'This comprehensive self-help book on all forms of anxiety during pregnancy and the year after birth is a must-read for women with anxiety problems during this period (clinicians are likely to find it a helpful resource too!). This up-to-date evidence-based resource, written by leading perinatal psychologists using cognitive-behavioural principles, includes consideration of how to cope with excessive worries about pregnancy and becoming a mother, needle phobia, pandemic-related anxieties, panic attacks, fear of childbirth, bonding concerns and more. Women will welcome its non-judgemental, supportive and wise words, and the self-help exercises in every chapter. If you fear you will not be able to cope with anxiety in the perinatal period this really is the book for you!'

Professor Louise M Howard
NIHR Research Professor in Women's Mental Health and NIHR Senior Investigator
Section of Women's Mental Health, Institute of Psychiatry, Psychology and Neuroscience, King's College London

'Having a baby is undoubtedly one of the most powerful experiences of life. Alongside joyful emotions, it is understandable that it may lead to more upsetting ones as well and most people are now aware of the possibility of post-natal depression. This book addresses the less discussed, but more common, impact of significant anxiety problems surrounding pregnancy, childbirth and early parenting. It lays out, with admirable clarity, the different forms this anxiety might take and provides guidance for how to deal with each of these, based on established cognitive behavioural principles. The book maintains a straightforward and compassionate approach, wearing its expertise lightly. It will be invaluable to all parents, whether it is your first child or a later one, and offers both the hope and practical advice we all need to break free from anxiety at this precious time.'

Nick Grey
Consultant Clinical Psychologist, Sussex Partnership NHS Foundation Trust

Break Free from Maternal Anxiety

Severe anxiety affects a huge number of women in pregnancy and the post-natal period, making a challenging time even more difficult. You may be suffering from uncontrollable worries about pregnancy and birth, distressing intrusive thoughts of accidental or deliberate harm to the baby, or fears connected to traumatic experiences. This practical self-help guide provides an active route out of feeling anxious. Step-by-step, the book teaches you to apply cognitive behavioural therapy (CBT) techniques in the particular context of pregnancy and becoming a new parent in order to overcome maternal anxiety in all its forms. Working through the book you will gain understanding of your anxiety and how factors from the past and present may be playing a role in how you feel. Together with practical exercises and worksheets to move through at your own pace, you will gain the tools you need to help you move forward and enjoy parenthood.

Dr Fiona Challacombe is a Lecturer in Perinatal Psychology in the Section of Women's Mental Health at the IOPPN, King's College London and a Clinical Psychologist at the Centre for Anxiety Disorders & Trauma, Maudsley Hospital, South London & Maudsley NHS Trust.

Dr Catherine Green is a Consultant Clinical Psychologist, Perinatal Mental Health Service, South West London and St Georges Mental Health NHS Trust.

Dr Victoria Bream is a Consultant Clinical Psychologist at the Oxford Health Specialist Psychological Interventions Clinic & Oxford Cognitive Therapy Centre, Oxford Health NHS Foundation Trust.

Break Free from Maternal Anxiety

A Self-Help Guide for Pregnancy,
Birth and the First Postnatal Year

Fiona Challacombe

King's College London

Catherine Green

South West London and St Georges Mental Health NHS Trust

Victoria Bream

Oxford Health NHS Foundation Trust

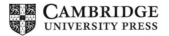
CAMBRIDGE
UNIVERSITY PRESS

CAMBRIDGE
UNIVERSITY PRESS

University Printing House, Cambridge CB2 8BS, United Kingdom

One Liberty Plaza, 20th Floor, New York, NY 10006, USA

477 Williamstown Road, Port Melbourne, VIC 3207, Australia

314–321, 3rd Floor, Plot 3, Splendor Forum, Jasola District Centre,
New Delhi – 110025, India

103 Penang Road, #05–06/07, Visioncrest Commercial, Singapore 238467

Cambridge University Press is part of the University of Cambridge.

It furthers the University's mission by disseminating knowledge in the pursuit of education,
learning, and research at the highest international levels of excellence.

www.cambridge.org
Information on this title: www.cambridge.org/9781108823135
DOI: 10.1017/9781108913539

© Cambridge University Press 2023

First published 2023

Printed in the United Kingdom by TJ Books Limited, Padstow, Cornwall

A catalogue record for this publication is available from the British Library.

Library of Congress Cataloging-in-Publication Data
Names: Challacombe, Fiona, editor.
Title: Break free from maternal anxiety : a self-help guide for pregnancy,
birth and the first postnatal year / Fiona Challacombe, King's College,
London, Catherine Green, South West London and St Georges Mental Health
NHS Trust, Victoria Bream, Oxford Health NHS Foundation Trust.
Description: Cambridge, United Kingdom ; New York, NY, USA : Cambridge
University Press, 2023. | Includes bibliographical references.
Identifiers: LCCN 2022002344 | ISBN 9781108823135 (paperback)
Subjects: LCSH: Anxiety. | Pregnancy–Psychological aspects–Popular works.
| Childbirth–Psychological aspects–Popular works. | Postpartum
depression–Popular works. | Mental illness in pregnancy–Popular works.
| BISAC: MEDICAL / Mental Health
Classification: LCC RG560 .B725 2023 | DDC 618.7/6–dc23/eng/20220329
LC record available at https://lccn.loc.gov/2022002344

ISBN 978-1-108-82313-5 Paperback

To MSA, IKCA & MKCA;
Stephen, Sophie and Toby;
Ian, SPO, BMB & SBB

Contents

About the Authors

We are all Chartered Clinical Psychologists and Accredited Cognitive Behaviour therapists working in the NHS. We have extensive experience in helping people overcome their anxiety disorders, often after they have made many unsuccessful attempts in the past. We contribute to academic research to improve the understanding of anxiety disorders and the effectiveness of treatments available. We are all mothers.

Dr Fiona Challacombe, Lecturer in Perinatal Clinical Psychology, King's College London & Lead Clinician, Parents with Anxiety Service, Centre for Anxiety Disorders & Trauma, South London and Maudsley NHS Trust

Dr Cathy Green, Consultant Clinical Psychologist, Perinatal Mental Health Service, South West London and St George's Mental Health NHS Trust

Dr Victoria Bream, Consultant Clinical Psychologist, Oxford Health Specialist Psychological Interventions Clinic, Warneford Hospital, Oxford; Oxford Cognitive Therapy Centre

How to Use This Book

You may be reading this book because you currently feel anxious, or because you think you might become anxious when you are pregnant or have a young baby, perhaps because of having had a tough time with anxiety in the past. Gaining a good understanding of what perinatal anxiety is, the different forms it can take, and the thought and behavioural patterns that can intensify it, can help you keep anxiety to a minimum and successfully navigate pregnancy and the postnatal period.

Where to Go First

There are many forms of anxiety with unique features to each, but there are also lots of common ideas that apply across all of them. Therefore, if you can, read the whole book. Alternatively, to find the chapters that will help you the most:

What is anxiety and how does it all work	Chapter 1: Introduction
I'm worrying and constantly thinking 'what if ... ', feeling uncertain and finding it difficult to make decisions	Chapter 2: Worry
I'm having horrible thoughts (or images or urges) that I wish I didn't have about bad things that I don't want to happen	Chapter 3: Intrusive Thoughts
I am terrified of being sick	Chapter 4: Phobias
I am terrified of blood or needles or pass out when I encounter them	Chapter 4: Phobias
I feel intense extreme panic out of the blue	Chapter 5: Panic

I have panic attacks or feel very worried about my health	Chapter 5: Panic
I avoid situations with other people and / or feel very anxious about social situations	Chapter 6: Social Anxiety
I have to get things exactly right and to a very high standard	Chapter 6: Perfectionism
I have had bad experiences that still affect me day to day	Chapter 7: Trauma
I am very fearful of childbirth	Chapter 8: Pregnancy-specific Anxiety
I am very anxious during my pregnancy	Chapter 8: Pregnancy-specific Anxiety
I am worried about becoming a parent	Chapter 9: Transition to Motherhood & Chapter 10: Applying Your Skills to Parenting

Maternal mental health and well-being is beginning to get the higher profile that it deserves, and there is more support and help available than ever before. You may have read books or online articles that have helped you feel understood or less alone when you are feeling stressed, worried or frightened. This is important, and this validation can be very helpful for many women.

If you want your feelings of anxiety to **change**, then this is the book for you. Cognitive behaviour therapy (CBT) is the recommended treatment for anxiety problems and we explain how to use the principles and specific strategies of CBT to help you to overcome this problem in all its forms. This is an *active* route out of feeling anxious. The suggestions are simple but very effective, and are based on decades of research around the world into using CBT for anxiety. This book will show you how to apply them in the particular context of pregnancy and becoming a new parent. In each chapter we aim to give you an understanding of how each form of anxiety affects women at this time, how factors from the past and present may be playing a role and how to use this understanding to move forward.

Whether your difficulties are an occasional annoyance or are very severe and interfere with most aspects of your life, this book can help you understand what is going on and work out how to start making changes to claim your life back and enjoy this period of pregnancy and beyond.

Please note:

Throughout the book we use case examples to illustrate how the different types of anxiety can affect people and what to do to move forward. We have constructed them to be useful and relevant, and representative of the mums that we work with in our NHS clinics, but they are not real individuals.

Within the book we refer to women and mothers. This is not intended to exclude birthing people of any gender or family configuration. We recognise there are many experiences and perspectives that are not represented in our writing but we hope the ideas will still prove helpful, however you identify and whatever your parenting journey. We also acknowledge that the experiences of fathers and partners is often overlooked and deserves attention in its own right. Many of the ideas and exercises may still be helpful for partners, or at the very least promote understanding of what you might be experiencing, and what they can do to help.

At the end of the book you will find a list of other useful resources and organisations that may be of help if you want to explore a particular issue further.

What This Book Is Not

This book is not a substitute for detailed and personalised medical or psychiatric assessment and guidance – please always follow the advice given to you by your midwife, doctor, and other qualified health professionals who know the specifics of your health and pregnancy. If you are seeking more support with your mental health, ask those involved in your care for a local referral and see our resources section for more information on getting help.

Acknowledgements

Our greatest thanks go to all the people we meet who experience anxiety and trauma, and who show great courage in overcoming their difficulties.

Many thanks to our past and present colleagues at the Centre for Anxiety Disorders and Trauma, South London & Maudsley NHS Foundation Trust, and the Oxford Health Specialist Psychological Interventions Clinic & Oxford Cognitive Therapy Centre. We are indebted to our colleagues Laura Bridle, Florence Bristow, Nick Grey, Louise Howard, Rachel Mycroft, and Kyla Vaillancourt.

This book would not have been possible without the support of our families and friends – particular heartfelt thanks to Maggie Green and Clare Hepworth.

1

• • • • • • •

Introduction

In this chapter you will learn:

➤ Why it is normal to feel anxious during pregnancy and after having a baby

➤ How to recognise what happens when you feel anxious

➤ The principles of a cognitive-behavioural understanding of maternal anxiety that underpin this book

➤ Why anxiety in pregnancy and motherhood is important to address for mums and babies

---

Why Is It Normal to Feel Anxious During Pregnancy and After Having a Baby, and When Is It a Problem?

The time of pregnancy and after having a baby can be very positive and exciting, but we know that it can also be challenging in lots of ways and mental health difficulties are common during pregnancy and postnatally. Contrary to popular belief, the most prevalent problem is anxiety rather than depression. In fact, about 15% of women will experience a significant anxiety problem at some point during pregnancy or the first postnatal year [1]. The high prevalence of anxiety during this time makes a lot of sense. The journey to, through and beyond pregnancy is paved with new experiences, uncertainty and unpredictability, all of which can generate or amplify feelings of anxiety. On top of this the stakes can feel especially high as you face new responsibilities of growing, birthing and caring for a baby. The general stress of sleep deprivation and physical, emotional and financial changes all play a role. Some women will adjust well to these new conditions, but for many others this process does not occur so readily. Anxiety is a normal emotion that is triggered in all of us from time to time, but an anxiety problem is said to occur when anxiety is excessive, persistent and interferes with aspects of your life.

Anxiety and feeling low often go hand in hand. Depression, a persistent feeling of low mood or loss of enjoyment in things, can make it hard to function. If you are experiencing depression or have been diagnosed with postnatal depression, this book could be useful to consider how the different stresses associated with pregnancy and becoming a parent are affecting you and what you can do about them. Many women we work with have low mood as a result of their anxiety problems, and getting on top of these can also help their mood lift. Sometimes this is not enough, and depression is a problem in its own right. More specific resources for treating depression are signposted at the end of this book.

What Is Anxiety?

Is my baby moving enough?
Will my baby be healthy?
Will I cope with the birth?
Will I be a good enough parent?
What will people think if he cries?
What if I drop her?

Just about every mother that has ever walked the planet has experienced anxious thoughts like these at some point. They aren't pleasant or comfortable and they certainly aren't spoken about enough, but they are a near universal part of pregnancy and parenthood. In fact, recent research has shown that 100% of new mothers experience intrusive, unwanted thoughts about something bad happening to their newborn in the first weeks after birth.

So, if you feel anxious, nervous or apprehensive in some way as a mum to be or a new mum, the first key message we want you to take away is **you are not alone.**

Of course, anxiety is not just a common aspect of motherhood but a normal part of being human and something most of us will be familiar with long before we begin our journey to being a parent. For example, when facing an exam, an important meeting or job interview, a big family occasion, public speaking or waking to hear a noise in the night. In certain circumstances, any of these situations could trigger a cascade of responses – body sensations, thoughts, images or memories that flash through our mind, feelings of fear and worry, alongside urges to respond in a certain way. We may not always be fully aware of all of them, but these quick, automatic signals have evolved over millions of years to help alert us to potential danger and ready our body for action to stay safe.

Our capacity for anxiety means we pay attention to danger, and this can be lifesaving – if this wasn't the case we probably wouldn't exist for very long and humans would have died out long ago! Consider the situation of crossing the road after meeting up with a friend. You hear the rev of an engine as you step out from the pavement. Without anxiety your brain wouldn't get the signals it needs to surge adrenaline, switch on the 'fight, flight or freeze' response and instantly escape the threat – in this case pulling quickly back onto the curb.

In basic evolutionary terms we have two main tasks as humans: survival and reproduction. It is very likely then that this hard-wired anxiety has given us an evolutionary advantage as it has helped us survive being eaten by predators and reproduce successfully.

 KEY IDEA

Anxiety is an essential part of being human that has enabled us to survive.

So, anxiety can be helpful, it has a purpose and has ensured the survival of our species. But unfortunately, it is not always accurate or useful. Any of us who have felt persistent anxiety will recognise it can also be unpleasant, uncomfortable and upsetting. It can stop us from doing the things we want to do and suck the fun out of life, including motherhood.

What Happens When We Feel Anxious?

Anxiety affects our minds, bodies, what grabs our attention and our behaviour. In this section we will consider this in more detail, so you can start to recognise the patterns that can occur.

An Anxious Mind

Our minds are rarely quiet – at any one time our thoughts might be full of words, pictures, memories from the past or a combination of some or all of these things. These might be positive, negative or neutral thoughts. Anxiety influences the content: when anxious, our minds typically churn up thoughts that are focused on negative things which might happen in the future – trying to predict if something 'bad' could happen, the worst-case scenarios, the potential danger ahead. We might have lots of 'what if … ' type thoughts, frightening images or memories of bad things that have happened to us. Our anxious mind can feel like a spotlight shining a light on our deepest fears, the problems we are facing now or in the future, or the potential danger around us.

Our relationships with others are also really important, so we are also sensitive to social threats. Anxious thoughts can also be judgements about ourselves, worries about what others are thinking, doubts about what we have or haven't done, or urges telling us what we 'should' or 'must' do thrown in for good measure. All of these 'thoughts' are quick fire, automatic and can leave us feeling worried, stressed, panicked, fearful or with a sense of dread. To make things worse, once we start feeling anxious, we are more likely to read into ambiguous or neutral situations as threatening or dangerous.

It would be impossible to list all the anxious thoughts that can occur, but here are some common ones women have talked about with us in pregnancy and after birth:

Thoughts

- *My baby isn't safe*
- *My baby isn't moving enough*
- *I won't cope with the birth*
- *What if I am not a good enough parent?*
- *What if she chokes?*
- *What if I drop the baby?*
- *What if that toy isn't clean?*

Images

- *Flashbacks to a previous birth*
- *Flashbacks to my own childhood*
- *Falling down the stairs with my baby*
- *Me abusing my baby*
- *Someone else harming my baby*

Judgements

- *I'm going mad*
- *I can't cope with parenthood*
- *I shouldn't feel this way about my baby*
- *Other people are angry because she's crying*

Doubts

- *Was he breathing?*
- *Did I make a mistake having a baby?*
- *Did I fasten the car seat?*
- *Did the steriliser really work?*

Urges

- *To throw my baby at the wall*
- *To make sure everything in the house is a certain way*

Anxiety will draw you into the content of the thought, but if you spend some time observing how your mind works when you feel anxious, you might also start to notice certain patterns or 'styles' in your thinking that aren't helping you to feel better. Some common patterns that are often linked to many forms of anxiety in the perinatal period are listed in the following section.

'Thinking the Worst'

Your anxious mind might jump to the worst-case scenario even though the initial problem or situation you are facing is quite small. This might be in the form of a verbal thought, e.g. a pain in your groin might trigger the thought 'The pain of childbirth will be unbearable', or you might spot an image or 'flash forward' to a future feared outcome. These attention-grabbing thoughts can elbow all the other possibilities out of the way.

'All or Nothing' or 'Black and White' Thinking

Here we mean a tendency to think in extremes, e.g. 'If it is not 100% right then I have failed'; 'I am either completely safe or in total danger'; 'if things are uncertain then they will go wrong'; 'if I don't achieve a vaginal birth then I am a total failure as a mother'. Anxiety can mean we take an overly rigid view of a situation that then gets in the way of seeing how the world really works – i.e. that there are often many shades of grey and life operates on a continuum rather than in extremes.

'Shoulds' and 'Musts'

Here we mean putting unreasonable (sometimes impossible) expectations or demands on yourself (or others), e.g. 'I should feel nothing but positive feelings about the prospect of motherhood'; 'I must eliminate *all* risk'; 'I shouldn't feel this overwhelmed – there must be something wrong with me'. This style of thinking is common amongst people who have a general tendency to set themselves high standards or strive for perfection.

Unsurprisingly it leads to feelings of stress and pressure and of course self-criticism when you fail to meet the standard.

Rumination or 'Post-mortems'

When you are anxious, it is natural to look for or spot evidence that fits with how you are feeling. This can mean churning over past experiences and conversations around pregnancy, birth or events that confirm to us we are in danger or we (or others) aren't capable or competent enough to ensure a positive outcome. This process naturally turns the temperature up on anxiety because it means we end up with rather 'tunnel vision' and only pay attention to a limited part of the picture.

Worry

By worry we mean the process of repeated negative thinking, usually in the form of sentences that start with 'What if ... '. You might be trying to feel more in control by running through various possibilities to 'plan for the worst' or you might feel that worrying in advance helps you to prevent something bad from happening or find solutions to problems. Alternatively, you might feel that worry controls you and there is nothing you can do to manage it. The tricky thing is that the more you engage in the process of churning worries in your mind, the more anxious you will feel. Worry itself doesn't solve problems or create more certainty or control – in fact it usually only fuels more doubt and discomfort.

Magical Thinking

Sometimes we might think of this as 'superstitious thinking' or a tendency to see two unrelated events as directly linked. This type of thinking is influenced by culture and society, but it is found in some form in all of them. In pregnancy, the idea of 'tempting fate' is a good example: you might think that by doing something, e.g. talking about your pregnancy before 12 weeks or buying things for your baby is 'risky' and that something bad might happen to the baby. The unfortunate reality is you can't eliminate risk in this way. Trying to do so often drives up anxiety as it keeps you focused on negative outcomes.

Emotional Reasoning

This is the idea that because we feel anxious, there must be something to be anxious about. However, sometimes, such as in the case of phobias for example, our threat system is activated when there is no threat, so this reasoning is very circular.

An Anxious Body

Anxiety is very physical. It is the body's alarm system and it is *very* effective. A stress response is triggered when we perceive a threat, and parts of our brain and a part of our nervous system called the 'sympathetic' or 'autonomic' nervous system kick into gear. When this happens, a brain structure called the amygdala sends signals to another part of our brain – the hypothalamus. This in turn sends signals to the pituitary gland which sits just below it in the brain. The pituitary gland releases a hormone telling our adrenal glands (which sit just above our kidneys) to release a flood of the hormones adrenaline, noradrenaline and cortisol into the body. This chain reaction is sometimes called your 'fight, flight or freeze' response. It is through the release of these hormones that rapid physical responses in the body occur, designed to help us protect ourselves. These are automatic and outside of our control. They are harmless but can feel very uncomfortable and sometimes frightening. Almost every organ in our body is affected.

Heart rate, breathing and blood pressure increase. This means we can move oxygen and other nutrients more quickly to our muscles and brain so we are able to face the danger or run away quickly. Our brains also prioritise survival functions. Blood is redirected from non-essential organs like our gut to our muscles, brain and heart. Feeling sick, having 'butterflies' in your tummy, appearing pale or flushed, feeling cold and clammy or hot and sweaty are all a result of this shift in blood flow. Our senses sharpen so we are in tune with our surroundings and vigilant for threat – for example our pupils dilate to take in more light so we can see clearly but this might mean we feel jumpy and on edge and it can be hard to concentrate on anything but the danger we perceive. Our muscles also tighten, leaving us tense and restless. Have a look at the table below for some more examples.

Part of the body	What is happening	Physical sensations we might notice
Heart and blood vessels	Heart rate increases Blood pressure increases Blood vessels dilate Blood redirected to brain and muscles – oxygen and nutrients circulate to the parts of the body where they are needed more quickly	Racing heart Hot Sweaty
Muscles	Increased blood flow, tightening	Tense, restless, on edge
Lungs	Breathing rate increases and airways dilate – more oxygen enters our blood	Breathless Tightness in the chest Dizziness
Skin	Perspire to cool our body down	Cold and clammy Hot and sweaty Hairs stand on end

The tricky thing is this alarm system is so efficient it kicks in when we face real danger but also when we *think* there is a danger (but there actually isn't). If you think of what it's like to watch a horror film or go on a roller coaster, you may recognise some of the sensations too. Think of it a bit like a faulty smoke alarm going off repeatedly even if there is no fire, for example when you burn toast or light a match. When that alarm is blaring it is hard to concentrate on what is actually happening and realise there is no real threat.

Anxious Reactions: Trying to Feel Safer

The point of anxiety is that it isn't pleasant and gets us to do things to try and resolve it. Naturally, we might feel pulled into action to try and feel safer and more in control. Our responses can include things we actively do, e.g. avoid, escape, check, seek reassurance, as well as things we try to do in our heads to feel better, e.g. churn over all potential scenarios or 'what ifs', ruminate, think positively, argue with ourselves and so on. They all have a purpose, but as we will discuss in detail throughout the book, can be counterproductive. Below are some examples of common 'safety-seeking strategies' you might adopt when you are feeling anxious.

What you do to try to feel safer	Example in pregnancy	Example post-birth
Avoidance	Avoiding any uncooked food	Avoiding talking about birth experience
Escape	Running out of a shop when feeling breathless	Leaving a parent group when the conversation turned to how sleep 'should' work for babies
Repeated checking or monitoring	Checking baby movements	Checking sleeping baby is breathing
Reassurance-seeking	Repeatedly looking online for the likelihood of chromosomal disorders	Repeatedly asking your partner if it's ok to feed the baby a particular food
Scanning for danger	Looking at and Googling ingredients for cleaning products	Repeatedly checking your baby for signs that they may be ill
Repeating a behaviour until you feel 'just right', e.g. handwashing	Handwashing when preparing a meal	Repeatedly fastening, undoing and refastening a car seat until it feels safe
Trying to suppress or control thoughts	Images of giving birth	Images of the delivery room

What you do to try to feel safer	Example in pregnancy	Example post-birth
Preparing for the worst (worry)	Thinking of all the ways pregnancy can 'go wrong'	Going out for a walk with every possible item required for every eventuality
Rumination / Post-mortems	Did I expose myself to contamination without knowing it?	Did I make a fool of myself in front of the other parents?
Mental checking	Trying to remember whether the baby moved in the same pattern as yesterday	Picturing whether I put the knives out of reach of the baby
Mental argument	I should be enjoying my pregnancy, is something wrong with me?	I know these thoughts are stupid, I should be able to ignore them

KEY IDEA

Anxiety affects our whole bodies, including what we think, feel and do.

Making Sense of Anxiety: A Cognitive-Behavioural Approach

Cognitive-behavioural theory is based on the idea that it's not just what happens in a particular situation, but *what we make of it* that affects how we feel and what we do. For example, if you say hello to a friend on the opposite side of the road and they walk on without waving back – you may think a number of things, including: 'Oh they didn't see me!', to 'Oh no, they don't like me', to 'Oh dear, they really need some glasses.' Each of these interpretations will connect with different moods and reactions.

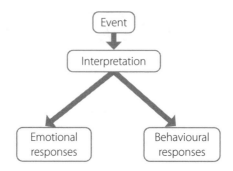

As you can see from this example, there are usually a number of possible ways to interpret an event, even when the event is very negative or even very positive; for example, experiencing a flashback of a road traffic accident and thinking 'I'm still thinking about this because I'm weak', or being at a very nice birthday party and thinking 'I'm not connecting with people even here because I'm weird'. The interpretation that most readily comes to mind is likely to be influenced by other experiences you have had, and your underlying beliefs about the world, yourself or other people. This explains why two people can experience similar events but have very different responses in terms of emotion and behaviour.

The responses themselves also play a very important role in the development of anxiety problems and what keeps them going. For example, considering the example of seeing your friend across the road, you may wave more vigorously at people the next time to make sure they see you, or alternatively decide not to wave at anyone again to avoid further perceived rejection. Each of these behaviours will in turn influence to some degree what then happens, and your further interpretations of the situation, including what you believe about yourself and others.

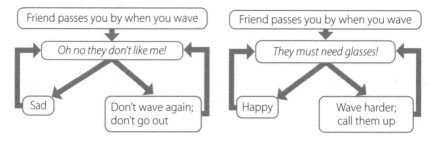

KEY IDEA

What we make of a situation influences our reactions, which can feed back into the interpretation.

The Perinatal Anxiety 'Equation'

Furthermore, anxiety is linked to our interpretations in particular ways. The severity of the anxiety you are experiencing will be a product of not just how *likely* you think something is, but how *awful* it would be for you personally if it happened, and how able you think you will be to cope with it, including whether you might get help from others.

Severity of anxiety about [EVENT] is proportional to:

$$\frac{\text{the likelihood of [EVENT] happening} \times \text{awfulness if X did happen}}{\text{how well I can cope} + \text{rescue} / \text{help from others}}$$

So even though we may realise something is not very likely, our anxiety is multiplied many times by our focus on how awful and difficult it would be if it *did* come true. This idea is relevant to all the anxiety problems we work with and explains why, when people give lots of reassurance, or people are told they need to try to 'be rational', it just doesn't work. Anxiety is an emotional problem. Pregnancy and birth are times of increased vulnerability to anxiety because there are all the key elements of any anxiety problem at a time of a very real increase in responsibility and uncertainty, lots of life changes as well as other stressors. It can really feel like it's all on you to resolve and solve all the issues related to the physical and mental health of your baby.

The important point is that, whilst these interpretations are usually very understandable, they may not be accurate, and they are changeable. You will learn a lot more about how to evaluate and challenge these ideas in relation to specific types of anxiety in the rest of this book.

Why Is Anxiety Important to Address in Pregnancy and Early Parenthood?

Excessive anxiety is, as you know, a horrible problem to have, at best taking the fun out of life but often taking away much more than that. Pregnancy and the postnatal period is of course very different to other times of life and it is normal to feel more risk-averse, vulnerable and careful. Even though the concept of 'normal' behaviour may be slightly different, it doesn't mean that you have to take *excessive* precautions relative to other women. Doing this can be highly stressful and impair your experience of pregnancy, birth and motherhood.

'Now' is always a good time to do something about it if you have an anxiety problem, but as you enter this new phase of life, making changes is likely not only to benefit you, but also those around you, including your baby. Being pregnant or a new mum means learning a lot of new skills and ways of being, so it is actually a particularly *good* time to tackle anxiety.

Is Anxiety Harmful for My Unborn Baby?

It is clear that the main person who is affected by anxiety is the person who is in the middle of it. Some studies of huge groups of women have highlighted a link between antenatal anxiety and stress and a raised chance of outcomes such as lower birth weight, earlier births or increases in emotional difficulties in children. This may sound frightening or upsetting but there are several important things to bear in mind – the overall rates of these things are relatively low [1]. The vast majority of mothers experiencing anxiety problems or any other issues or no anxiety do not have these outcomes. Often women coming to our clinics have heard or are told about these studies and pick up the message that they are somehow harming their baby just by being anxious, unfortunately leading to lots more worry for some. Remember that worrying and anxiety to some degree is very normal and unavoidable and of course helpful in some circumstances. The best any of us can do in pregnancy and beyond is to try and take care of ourselves and work on excessive anxiety. Doing this will have a big influence on your well-being and by extension theirs.

Is it Safe to Tackle Anxiety in Pregnancy?

Ironically, sometimes there are also unhelpful messages related to actually tackling anxiety in pregnancy. Pregnancy is a good time to tackle anxiety and the principles are just the same as outside this time. This involves first getting a good understanding, then applying this by testing things out and getting new knowledge and experiences. This process is sometimes called exposure, as you are 'exposing' yourself to your fears. A term we prefer and use in this book is behavioural experiments, or 'testing things out', because you are generally taking an informed approach to what you are testing out and why. Of course, doing something you have previously avoided may be a little anxiety-provoking at first, but this generally subsides. The experiments are not about going into extreme situations, but are about doing things that the *average* pregnant woman would do.

We are aware that occasionally women are told (sometimes by health professionals not trained in how to help people overcome anxiety), that doing exposure that could make them feel anxious during pregnancy could be harmful to their baby. This is not founded on evidence and is a good example of how the system around people can feed into the things that keep anxiety going. It rather misses the point that people are doing the exposure because they are *already* anxious! Secondly, although exposure tasks might initially raise anxiety, this quickly reduces and there is very good evidence that these kinds of exposure experiments lead to overall improvements in anxiety as people find out how the world really works and acclimatise to this new way of doing things, which is very much the idea of this approach [2].

We can therefore assume that working on anxiety can only help both mother and baby.

To Sum Up

- Anxiety problems are common – you are definitely not alone
- Anxiety itself is not dangerous even though it can make you *feel* in danger
- Anxiety makes pregnancy and being a parent even harder than it is already
- Anxious feelings occur at the same time as thoughts, doubts or images about bad things happening
- You can identify and change your anxiety-related thinking and the ways of managing anxiety which might not be helping you to feel better
- You *can* change how anxious you feel

2

• • • • • • •

Persistent and Distressing Worry

In this chapter you will learn:

➤ How to recognise a worry problem
➤ To understand in detail the processes and beliefs that keep worry going
➤ Techniques to practise in order to reduce worrying
➤ How to work out the difference between problem-solving and worrying
➤ How to reduce self-critical thinking

What Is a Worry Problem?

'Worrying' is generally used to describe repeatedly thinking about a future topic or occurrence, usually associated with feeling anxious and preoccupied. Everyone worries from time to time, especially parents. It is also common to hear the word 'worry' used to describe everyday minor preoccupations, e.g. 'I'm a bit worried that we might miss that train' or 'that bad weather forecast tomorrow is a bit of a worry'. These concerns will usually be fleeting and forgotten within hours. Problematic worry is when you get stuck in repeated loops of negative anxious thinking that feel hard to stop, control or turn away from. It can feel like a very rapid 'downward spiral' as the same thoughts churn over and over in your mind and the focus of your worry begins to loom larger and larger. It is one of the most common problems in pregnancy and postnatally, with about 8% of women experiencing problematic worry.

You might notice that you are thinking repeatedly about how things could go wrong or turn out badly and what might happen if this were to occur. You might think this helps you to mentally prepare and problem-solve but usually it just ends with feeling more anxious, unconfident and uncertain as your mind takes you around in circles or jumps to more and more 'worst-case scenarios', and a belief that you won't cope well.

A really key point therefore, is that *repeatedly* worrying is never helpful, even though it might feel that you are doing something in response to a problem. Solving problems, or thinking through and making decisions, is helpful but repeatedly thinking of future worst-case scenarios is distressing and does nothing to avoid or prevent bad things from actually happening. All that happens is you end up trapped inside your head with a sense of dread. This is likely to make it tricky to concentrate on other things. On top of this, repeated worrying can take up a lot of time and energy, make you feel physically tense and stop you sleeping well. None of which is terribly helpful if you are pregnant or trying to take care of a young baby.

Here are some examples of worries that might seem familiar. Very often we can spot worry as it starts with the question 'What if ... ?' before unfolding into a chain of negative thoughts:

What if the baby isn't getting enough milk?

What if I can't work out why the baby is crying and he cries all day?

I need to go to the shops, but I'm so tired, what if we have a car accident? How do I know if I'm fit to drive?

What if I do something that undermines or upsets one of the other mums in the group?

What if none of the other mums like me?

What if we are living in the wrong house?

When we go out, what if I can't fold the buggy or get it in the car?

What if I get made redundant?

Every new parent will think some of these kinds of thoughts from time to time, and these worries will be more or less bothersome depending on the amount of sleep you and your baby have had, what else is going on that day, and what else is going on in your life in general – if you have serious concerns about money, your relationships, your work situation, or your future plans it is natural that those things will be on your mind and add to overall feelings of stress and uncertainty. What we will focus on in this chapter is when worrying – asking yourself all these 'what if' questions – starts to take over and bother you even on a 'good day', and perhaps leads to you feeling very tense and stressed, not enjoying or avoiding situations [1].

Worrying in Pregnancy

Hestia

Hestia was 32 weeks pregnant. She constantly worried about every decision that she made about the baby, thinking 'What if I haven't included everything on my birth plan'; 'What if I buy the wrong buggy?'; 'Is it ok to get a second-hand high chair?'; 'What if I can't find a good school when the baby is older?'; 'What if I lose my job when I am on maternity leave?'.

Once she started thinking these thoughts, she found it very difficult to move her attention to other things. She noticed she was feeling very tense, was snappy and irritable with her partner, and unable to concentrate on her work, and struggled to stay focused when reading a book. Hestia felt so jumpy and nervous that she felt reluctant to go out and see friends or go to her pregnancy exercise class, and started taking days off work. She avoided making any decisions about the baby as she feared triggering more worries.

Even when Hestia was feeling quite happy and ok in other ways, she found it hard not to worry. Hestia's dad was 'a worrier', and there were family mottos such as 'If in doubt, don't' and 'Prepare for the worst because then at least it's a nice surprise when it goes well'. She didn't know whether to talk about these worries with her parents in case that worried them too.

Worrying Postnatally

Lissa

Lissa had a 16-week-old baby. She found it difficult when she couldn't be 100% certain about an aspect of her baby's care: 'Did he have enough sleep to make sure that he will keep growing?'; 'Was that enough milk for him to stay asleep for a few hours?'; 'What if he wakes up after a short sleep and I can't cope?'; 'Did he have enough tummy time?'; 'Is his head a strange shape?'. She found her worries jumped from one concern to another.

On top of her exhaustion due to night-time feeds, she found herself awake at night worrying about all sorts of different concerns about her baby and his future health and development, and her own life and whether it was going in the right direction. Other women in her family seemed to find motherhood easy, and didn't appear to have any of these doubts or worries. Lissa often told herself 'Don't be stupid' when she worried, and tried to get the worries out of her head. Sometimes she asked other family members for reassurance about her worries, and whilst they answered her questions kindly and offered to help when they could, she still worried. Sometimes she would check online for information about her worries, but this led to her worrying more.

OVER TO YOU
Is Worry a Problem for You?

Do you:

- Find yourself thinking over and over about things that could go wrong in the future?
- Often think 'But what if … and then what if … '?
- Have worries that jump from topic to topic?
- Usually think about the worst thing that could happen?
- Find it hard to stop worrying once you start?
- Feel apprehensive a lot of the time?
- Find it hard to focus or concentrate on things fully because of worry?

- Worry even when you are having a good day or feel generally happy or ok?
- Feel stressed, edgy, tense and anxious or irritable and snappy?
- Have difficulties getting to sleep or staying asleep because you are worrying?

Why It's a Good Idea to Tackle a Worry Problem

You may have heard 'Don't worry about that' or 'You worry too much' or 'There is nothing to worry about' from people around you, but persistent worry is not easy to just dismiss. Worrying excessively is not a trivial problem. However, it is important to work on reducing worry, as research studies have found that worrying is associated with increased depression in the later stages of pregnancy and postnatally. Repetitive worrying takes up a lot of mental energy and makes it very hard to live in the moment. It also makes it harder to solve problems and reduces confidence in problem-solving. If you imagine trying to perform a task whilst a disaster movie is playing in your head, this is not surprising. In a study about mums who were prone to high levels of worry, when researchers asked the mums to focus on their worries, they were more preoccupied and paid less attention to their babies. However, they *were* able to tune into their babies when they were not worrying [2].

Is This a Worry Problem or Another Kind of Anxiety?

Worry is a very widely used word in everyday conversation. In this chapter we are thinking about repetitive 'what if' worry, feeling apprehensive or stressed, and questioning your decisions – if you think your worries don't quite fit with what has been described so far, keep reading but also consider reading these other chapters:

If your worries are intrusive, unwanted thoughts, images or urges and you feel that you need to act on the thoughts to stop something bad happening	Chapter 3: Unwanted Intrusive Thoughts of Harm

If your repeated thoughts are about a past event where something bad or traumatic happened to you or someone you know	Chapter 7: Coping with Traumatic Experiences while Pregnant and after Birth
If your worries are about your physical health, and you worry that there is something seriously wrong with you	Chapter 5: Panic Attacks and Health Worries
You are worried about medical procedures such as blood tests or injections	Chapter 4: Specific Phobias Affecting Pregnancy and the Postnatal Period
You worry about specific aspects of pregnancy and birth a great deal, with few other topics of worry	Chapter 8: Anxiety about Pregnancy and Birth
You worry about getting things exactly right, all the time, and judge yourself on your 'performance'	Chapter 6: Feeling Anxious around Other People

Understanding How it Works: A Vicious Flower of Worry

Problematic worry sticks around as it entwines itself with all aspects of your thinking. When you are worrying you may:

- Perceive the world as more dangerous than it actually is
- Hold beliefs that worry is helping you – or that worry itself is dangerous
- Find it hard or impossible to cope with any uncertainty
- Do things or avoid things to try to feel less worried, but might actually make things worse
- Be harsh to and critical of yourself

Worry may have got the better of you for some time. It might be difficult to imagine that there is a way out of this problem as you may feel quite stuck and demoralised, or even believe that worry is helpful and stops bad things from happening. The good news is persistent worrying can be

How to work on worry

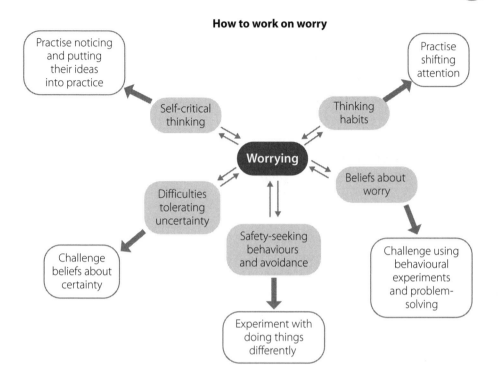

tackled and we aim to show you how. The 'vicious flower' diagram shows these aspects, and how you work on each petal.

What Makes the Worries So Hard to Dismiss: How You Interpret Situations and the Focus of Your Attention

Worrying is linked with how we respond to signals in the world around us. Research into worry shows that people who worry are more likely to interpret an ambiguous situation as a threat, e.g my baby makes a face when I give him a new food – 'What if it makes him ill?'. Whereas people who do not worry would interpret the same situation as neutral or positive, e.g. 'He must have never had this taste before' or 'What a funny face, he can't work out if he loves it or hates it' [3]. This tendency to interpret situations as negative can trigger further negative thoughts and start the worry process of repeatedly thinking about negative outcomes of future events. Research also shows that once you start worrying, threatening information grabs your attention – like a powerful spotlight focused on the potential bad outcome. Other information or perspectives are in the dark, and unseen, as the spotlight is difficult to shift.

OVER TO YOU
Why Can't I Stop Worrying?

Your thinking habits:

> If a situation is uncertain, how does your thinking tend to respond? Can you go ahead, unconcerned with the uncertainty, or do you find yourself trying to control or reduce uncertainty?
>
> Do you notice yourself jumping to a negative thought or outcome, and thinking 'what if' that happens?

If this is sounding familiar, remember that it is not your fault that you have started worrying and been drawn into this kind of thinking – once a worry problem starts, it takes on a life of its own. Cognitive behavioural therapy (CBT) focused on overcoming persistent worry has helped to find ways to tackle worry processes very specifically – you can't 'just stop worrying' if your thinking has become more tuned into noticing threatening information, and you see more threat or danger in situations than people who are not experiencing a worry problem. These are 'thinking habits' and it will be helpful to practise and rehearse doing things differently – we will go through these together.

What Makes the Worries So Hard to Dismiss: Beliefs About Worry

Your ideas about what worrying does or doesn't achieve are an important part of understanding why you might be having a hard time tuning out or turning away from worry. You might have a number of positive ideas about worry, e.g. 'Worry helps me to prepare'; 'Worry helps me solve problems'; 'Worry keeps me safe'; 'Worry will help me be certain', which naturally mean your mind pulls worry closer rather than allowing you to get out of your own thinking and on with your life. Alternatively, you might have a number of negative or more frightening thoughts about worry, e.g. 'Worry is dangerous for me and my baby – I'm going to get so stressed one or both of us will be harmed'; 'Worrying is uncontrollable and can't be stopped.'

OVER TO YOU
Identifying Beliefs About Worry

What do you see as the advantages to worrying?
What are the downsides or fears you have about worrying?

What Makes the Worries so Hard to Dismiss: Things You Do to Try to Feel Better but Keep the Worry Going

If you 'worry about worrying' in the way we describe above, you might try to do things to stop it – you might avoid situations for fear of triggering the worries, e.g. avoiding going out as you worry your baby may be unsettled, or you won't remember everything; you might try to push the worries out of your mind (only to find they bounce back) or zone out or dull the worries with alcohol or fiddling on your phone. You might find yourself arguing with yourself or telling yourself to 'just stop worrying, think positive!' or criticising yourself for 'being so ridiculous'. You might seek out reassurance or 'certainty' by checking things out with loved ones, overly planning and preparing, perhaps with a lot of lists to help you feel more in control, or over-researching topics of worry online. The tricky thing with all these strategies is they don't solve your anxiety as they only pull your attention back onto worry, undermine your confidence in yourself, lead to more doubt and uncertainty or feelings of overwhelm and prevent you from putting your beliefs about worry to the test.

OVER TO YOU
What Strategies Do You Use to Try and Stop or Control Worrying?

Do you avoid certain situations for fear of triggering worry? Which situations do you tend to avoid?

Do you argue with yourself or tell yourself to think differently?

Do you churn the worry over in the hope you will come to a more certain conclusion and be able to move on?

Do you try to distract yourself in some way? What do you do?

Do you make a lot of lists, or spend a lot of time planning, or over-prepare in an effort to feel more in control?

Do you do a lot of research online to try and feel more certain, but still feel unconfident about your decision?

Moving Forward: Tackling Your Anxiety-related Thinking

So far, we have not asked you to think much about what it is that you worry about (the content). That is because when you are working to change your worrying, *what* you are thinking about is less important than the *way* you are thinking about it (the process). You have probably noticed that you can worry about anything (or everything) and that very often the focus of your worry will jump from topic to topic very quickly. The theme or content of the worry could be anything, so we will not focus on trying to work out the specific content of your worry. Trying to challenge the content of your worry often just leads to feeling more tangled up in your head as you get stuck in a process of arguing with yourself. Unfortunately, worry is often about things we just cannot be sure of so the argument could literally never end! Instead, you will need to focus on solutions which tackle the way that worry works.

KEY IDEA

The problem is not what you worry about but the way you get stuck churning over the worrying thoughts.

Challenging the Belief: Worrying Helps Me Work Things Out and Is Helpful

Sometimes we need to actually solve a problem, and worrying does not help. Practise working this out.

Ask yourself:

1. Is this actually important? Will anyone else care about this tomorrow, or next year, or on their deathbed? Will I care about this on my deathbed?!

Let's take an example worry of 'what if I am late to meet my friends?' If you can step back and think about this, would your friends notice if you were late, or would they understand if you were a bit late, or perhaps several of them would be late themselves? Even if you inconvenience them for a short while, is it really that bad? How much of your time and effort is it worth to think about this? You don't have time or energy to spare, is it the best use of that time to go over and over what may or may not happen?

If you can consider the idea that this is not important, try to get on with what you are doing, and if your worries come back in, treat them as white noise in the background. Focus your attention on things that really do matter to you. The sections below on shifting your attention, worry times and tolerating uncertainty will help you.

If you consider that what you are worrying about is important, ask yourself:

2. Can I do something about this? Is this something I can influence, and is that within my control?

Let's take the example of a worry of 'my baby is six months old and I need to start weaning, but what if I can't do it?'

Step 1: define the problem: I need a plan for weaning

Step 2: generate as many solutions as possible:

Ask the health visitors at the baby clinic

Ask other mums

Buy a book on weaning

Look online for advice

Step 3: identify pros and cons of each option

	Pros	Cons
Ask the health visitors	They will give me up to date advice and some leaflets	They don't have much time to talk Sometimes the baby clinic is really busy and I want to get out of there as soon as possible
Ask other parents	Some of my friends have already offered to swap recipes and eat together	I might not want to do it the same way as them
Buy a book on weaning	A book will have meal plans and recipes that would give me some structure I could look in the library first and see if there were any good ones	I might not be able to decide which book to buy
Look online for advice	Some celebrities have really good websites with good tips; reading these usually makes me feel quite good as they are full of positive messages and practical ideas	There are lots of different sites and I might get overwhelmed with which one to stick to

Step 4: 'road test' your solution

Once you have picked an option, plan how you will carry out the solution to the problem.

Write yourself a note of what you need to do – be very specific, including when you can do it, and / or who you need to help you with it. E.g.:

I will look at the celebrity Joe Wicks's website and get five recipes from his weaning section.

I will do this at 6.30 pm tomorrow night. My partner finishes work at 6.15
pm – we have agreed that they will make me a cup of tea, then give the
baby a bath, and I will sit in the bedroom on my own for 15 minutes. After
10 minutes I will stop reading and write down / bookmark five recipes. If I
haven't finished reading, then I will still note the recipes.

Yes but … 'I Don't Have Time to Problem Solve'

It is not easy to dedicate time to these problems when you are pregnant or
looking after a young baby, but if you break it down into smaller steps, and
get other people to help you when you can, you will be in a better position
to approach it. Remember that worrying eats into your time, saps your
energy and undermines your confidence in yourself and your judgement.
If you can find five minutes whilst your baby is asleep, or engaged with a
toy, or being looked after by someone else, grab a pen and start writing on
whatever you can find – many great plans have been hatched on the back
of an envelope or a napkin!

Yes but … 'I Can't Stop Worrying About Whether I've Picked the Right Solution to the Problem'

If the worries are getting the better of you when you are trying to think of
what you can do, try approaching it as if someone else came to you with the
same problem, and write down what would you do to help them. Do you
think that everyone picks the right solution first time? If only – we all learn
things by trying different ideas and seeing which ones work best for us.

Finally, ask yourself:

3. Is this a worry about something that may or may not happen in the future,
and that is out of my control?

For example, what if there is another pandemic? What if my baby gets a serious illness when they are older? What if my baby has a learning difficulty
or developmental problem? What if I choose the wrong school and they get
bullied? What if interest rates go up and we cannot afford our mortgage?

Going over and over these kind of thoughts does not help, and will make you feel more anxious and preoccupied, and with less available attention and energy to deal with your day-to-day life. Getting out of this kind of worrying needs some active work on challenging your thinking – the rest of this chapter takes you through some simple but effective ways to get out of constant worry.

Moving Forward: Shifting Your Attention Away from Worry

At the start of this chapter, we described how when you are worrying, frightening or threatening information grabs your attention – like a powerful spotlight focused on the potential bad outcome. Other information or perspectives are in the dark, and the spotlight is difficult to shift. You may find it very hard to re-direct that spotlight beam onto something else. The best plan is to practise – like changing any habit, or learning any new skill, you will need to repeatedly practise spotting yourself worrying, and really try to engage your attention with the 'task at hand'. The good news is that you have a very engaging and attention-demanding person with you all the time – your yet to be born or new baby. You might be able to distract yourself sometimes by doing something different.

Let's consider how this would work for Hestia:

Hestia wanted to feel certain that she had made a good decision. She really struggled with any uncertainty, and usually spent a lot of time researching choices and thinking about the pros and cons of e.g. buying a particular product or where to go for a day out.

However, she had started to avoid decisions as she was getting weighed down in worry and thinking about how bad she would feel if she made the 'wrong' choice. For example, when thinking about buying a buggy, she feared that she would choose a particular model and then regret it, and that she would be ashamed of herself for not thinking it through 'properly' and that other people would think badly of her.

Hestia noticed herself worrying more later in the day when she was more tired and feeling physically wrecked. When she noticed the 'what if' thinking, or noticed her shoulders tightening, or tension in her neck, she deliberately moved her attention to her growing baby. She paid attention to the movements and sensations from her baby, and gave her attention to the wonder of pregnancy and to her soon-to-arrive baby.

She reminded herself that the baby would not be bothered about whether the buggy is the one that cost £1,000 or the one that cost £50, and that all that really mattered was that she was going to do her best to be a good mother. This was difficult to keep up, as she would think 'What if the baby isn't moving enough?', or 'What if the cheap buggy means the baby won't be able to lie flat enough?', or 'What if I can't cope with being a mother?'

It was hard, but Hestia practised that shift again, moving her focus to what else she was doing, focusing on the book she was reading, or the meal she was cooking, or how weird her toes felt now she was pregnant, and practised treating the worries as background noise. Over time she felt more in control of her worries, and less stressed and tense.

Challenging the Belief 'I Can't Stop Worrying' or 'My Worry Is Out of My Control'

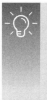 **KEY IDEA**

Worrying grabs your attention, and keeps you focused on negative possibilities. Practise deliberately moving your attention to what you are doing right now. This will become easier with practice.

If this was easy, you would have done this already. This is effortful. Don't be demoralised – you will have had to practise and try hard to learn other things in your life – and you managed it. Try to note your practice at shifting away from your worries over the next week – use a chart like this, or some post-it notes, or anything that helps you to note that you tried to do this, and to show that the more you practise, the more you can move your attention away from worries.

	Day 1	Day 2	Day 3	Day 4	Day 5	Day 6	Day 7
Practising shifting my attention spotlight from worries to what I am doing	✔✔	✔✔✔	✔✔✔✔	✔	✔✔✔✔	✔✔✔	✔✔✔✔✔✔
Difficulty	10/10 difficulty!	9/10	8/10	10/10	7/10	7/10	5/10

Worry-free Zones

Another way of approaching this is to set 'worry-free zones'. Make a conscious decision to put your worries to one side for a set time in the day, starting with a short slot in the day somewhere. It is up to you whether you link this to a particular task or time – maybe every time you have a much-needed snack to fuel your pregnant or postnatal body you can try to focus away from worry and enjoy every second of your crisps or chocolate, or if you hear a nineties hit on the radio – take that time to enjoy the track and put your worries to one side. You might decide that a particular time of day is your break from worrying – maybe first thing in the morning. This may sound too simple, but this is a well-used technique in CBT for worry problems. Your worries keep popping in, and you can keep practising that shift – remember to be kind to yourself, and not beat yourself up if you have a day when you can't seem to do this at all. Over time, as you get more practice, you can try to increase the worry-free zones. You are changing your relationship with your worrying thoughts – rather than the thoughts dominating your thinking, you are exercising control over the worry process.

Yes but … Isn't All This Just Distracting Myself? That Doesn't Work for Me as I End Up Worrying Again

What you are practising is the *shift* from worry to something else, rather than finding a distraction. It doesn't matter what you use as your prompt to make the shift, the idea is to identity something that reminds or prompts you to engage in that active move of your focus from worries to what you are doing in that moment – it doesn't matter if your 'task in hand' is eating crisps or reading a book on brain surgery, so long as you are practising that shift, you are working on your worry problem.

Planning a Worry Time

Another approach from what we know about how CBT can help with worry is to plan a time when you *will* worry, and deliberately postpone worrying until that specific time. This might seem strange, but this is a useful strategy to free yourself from the relentless worrying, by setting a particular time when you can come back to worries you have noted in the day. Finding a set time of day might be difficult when you are looking after a newborn, so you might need to experiment with how to make this work, e.g. one 15-minute slot at some point between 1–3 pm.

> Lissa decided that every time she put her baby on the floor to have a wriggle, she would refocus her attention to her baby, and away from her worries. She looked at her baby's facial expression and how the baby was moving, and enjoyed seeing her baby trying out new moves on the mat. She noticed worries coming back in ('what if the baby doesn't ever roll? Should she be wearing those tight socks? Will her head get really flat if I leave her here too long?') and felt anxious and very sad. She got up and kept talking to her baby whilst she made a cup of tea and got a large flapjack. She reminded herself that she was only human, and that she was finding it hard not to worry but she was working on it. She sat back down with her baby and refocused on her 'worry-free zone'; she enjoyed watching the wriggling and having a few minutes to drink her tea and get her energy levels back up.

Moving Forward: Dealing with Uncertainty

Feeling uncertain is a difficult feeling, and we all try to feel sure and certain about aspects of our lives. When worry becomes a problem, a big trap is believing that worrying makes things more certain and predictable. Sadly, worry makes you feel bad, takes up your time and energy, and keeps you focused on negative outcomes and scenarios.

OVER TO YOU
Accepting (Some) Uncertainty

Have a think about these questions:

Have you ever had a time in your life when you have been certain about everything? Has anyone? Is being 100% certain possible in any situation in your life at the moment?

Can you think of any examples when you were able to accept being uncertain?

What are the costs of trying to be certain?

Has worrying about things made you more certain? Or less?

Has worrying about things made things more predictable?

For uncertain situations, have you spent a lot of time focused on the bad outcome rather than other possibilities? Has this helped you? What was the cost of this?

There is no magic fix that makes you suddenly able to be really relaxed about uncertainty or predictability. Other people who are less prone to worry may have told you to 'relax, don't worry about it,' which is unlikely to have helped. What will help is recognising that worry is not helping you, and being courageous and accepting some uncertainty, reducing your efforts to try to be certain.

Sitting with Uncertainty Instead of Trying to Solve It

If you would like to build up your tolerance of uncertainty, a first step is to begin to notice the need for it. Can you spot the struggle, the urge to do something to try and be sure, the discomfort with feeling doubts, how it is making you feel emotionally and physically? For example:

> *I notice how much I am struggling right now not to be absolutely certain my baby will be born healthy.*

> *I notice my need for a guarantee and how anxious and agitated that makes me feel.*

> *I feel hot and tense and have a very strong urge to ask for more reassurance from my husband or call my midwife so I can try and escape this feeling but I know they can't give me any cast iron guarantees.*

Next can you experiment with accepting the uncertainty here? Can you resist the urge to seek certainty either by overthinking or seeking reassurance in some way? If that feels too difficult, could you postpone acting on that urge for a few minutes and try and turn your attention onto something else that can occupy you for a while or ask for support (e.g. a hug) instead of reassurance? For example:

> *I know my need for certainty can't be satisfied right now and I also know a range of outcomes are possible. I know trying to be sure in some way right now only keeps me preoccupied and anxious and doesn't give me what I need. I will do my best not to ask for reassurance, accepting that this is an uncertain situation I have to sit with. I will try to turn my attention onto something else that I enjoy – I might put some music on or call a friend.*

For some more tips on tackling reassurance seeking specifically, see Chapter 3 on unwanted intrusive thoughts.

American psychologists Michel Dugas and Melisa Robichaud are experts in understanding worry. They worked with many people with worry problems who found it difficult, or intolerable, to have any uncertainty. They used the idea of having a 'psychological allergy' to uncertainty, as even a tiny bit of uncertainty can provoke a huge and distressing reaction. If you believe that being uncertain is impossible to tolerate, or will lead to bad things happening, you can test out these ideas. This is how it would work for Lissa:

> Lissa wanted to go out more with her baby, but struggled to get out of the door as she kept on thinking about what she might need, and whether she would be prepared. She thought: 'I need to know, I need to be certain otherwise everything will go wrong. I must plan for everything, I don't want to be 'taken by surprise' when I'm out as I will be paralysed, very anxious and the baby will be inconsolable, which will be my fault.'

Before the experiment		After the experiment	
Planned experiment (what / where / when)	What are you testing out, what do you predict will happen (and how believable is it)?	What happened?	How does the world really work?
Go out with nappies, wipes and nothing else	Something will happen and I will not be prepared I will be very anxious (100% anxiety for the whole time) The baby will cry for an hour and I will not be able to soothe him (100%)	I did feel 100% anxious as I left the house and I nearly went back. I was crying. Once I got out, I walked past the shops and something made the baby very excited and he was really kicking his legs – I stopped to see what it might be, and this made me happy, seeing him engage with the outside world We stayed out for an hour and a half, and he did grizzle a little after half an hour, but he was filling his nappy. Once I changed him, he was ok again. So he didn't get really upset, and I was able to look after him and soothe him	It is possible to go out with only a few things and for everything to be ok – I believe this 50/50. I need to keep practising to feel more convinced that I can go out without having absolutely everything I need for all possible eventualities

OVER TO YOU

Work Out Your Antidote to Your Intolerance of Uncertainty Allergy

Think how this would work for you – what is the worst thing about being uncertain for you? How can you do something that gives you some evidence from real-world experience, rather than being caught in the endless loops of worry and horrible feelings of anxiety?

Before the experiment		After the experiment	
Planned experiment (what / where / when)	What is the anxious prediction (and how believable is it)?	What happened?	How does the world really work?

Moving Forward: Tackling Self-critical Thinking

During pregnancy and throughout parenting, there are endless opportunities to think that you are getting it 'wrong' or 'failing'. Just like the worry thoughts, or like the unwanted intrusive thoughts detailed in Chapter 3, it is really important to practise disregarding self-critical thoughts, as they will fuel your anxiety and make you feel miserable. If you are frequently putting yourself down, calling yourself names, and have a low opinion of yourself, you can help yourself to build up a fairer, kinder view of yourself that is based on reality. Acknowledging your positive qualities and being compassionate to yourself will not turn you into an arrogant or egotistical person – it will help you to enjoy being a parent and protect you from the ups and downs that are inevitable in this new chapter of your life.

Imagine you were at a good friend's house, and another person barged into the room, and started saying to your friend: 'You're rubbish at this, you're a loser, you're hopeless, you don't get anything right, you can't even make a cup of tea properly, everyone else can do this, what's wrong with you?' Probably you would get up and eject that person from the room, make it clear to them they were never to return, and comfort your friend, telling them that the person had no right to say any of those things, and they shouldn't believe a word of it. If you have a constant critic like this in your head, it won't make you better at what you are trying to do, or make you happy or fulfilled, unfortunately it will do the opposite.

Self-critical thinking can become a habit and can feel difficult to stop. You can do several things to steer yourself away from self-critical thinking. Dr Melanie Fennell is an expert in overcoming critical thinking and promoting healthy self-esteem. She has developed self-help materials that have been read by hundreds of thousands of people – so if this is something you need, it's not just you. See the resources sections for details of her book. If you have read other chapters in this book, you will have read that one of the useful places to start with any problem is to catch it happening. With self-critical thoughts, it is a useful exercise to re-examine the thought, and judge whether it is a fair and reasonable way to evaluate yourself as a person. You can try and think of alternative statements about yourself that also focus on all your strengths. Finally, put this into practice – get up and out and try out these different ideas about yourself; see the example below.

Catch it	Write down what you are thinking when you feel particularly anxious or upset, or any other strong negative emotion	Upset when I saw other pregnant mums going into a yoga class when I was going to work 'Already I'm not a good enough mum'
Re-examine it	Is there any evidence against the self-critical thought? Would I say this about another person in the same circumstances? Am I focused only on things that are not going well and ignoring things that are ok or good?	Not all mums go to yoga, or even like yoga; just because I'm not doing it doesn't mean that I don't care about my health or the baby Yoga does not = good mum! I'd say to someone else to do what they want to do and not get dragged into ticking off a list of what they think they should be doing

Alternative	What could I conclude is a fairer and more accurate way to think about myself? How would a good friend or a family member I get on with describe me? How would a colleague describe me?	I'm doing well with lots of aspects of being a mum. I am working so that I have enough money to take maternity leave for a longer period. I am walking to work to get some exercise. I have a packed lunch that is both delicious and good for me. I have attended all my antenatal checks and I have looked after my health
Put it into practice	What can I do to get out of this self-critical thinking?	Write down what I have done well, no matter how small

Yes but … I'm Going to Feel Really Lame Writing Down 'I Made Dinner and It Was Nice'

(1) Well done on making a nice dinner whilst pregnant or caring for a little baby – it didn't arrive by magic, and (2) you will not have to do this for the rest of your life! You need to do it for a relatively short time to shift your thinking (back) to treating yourself fairly, and to get out of the habit of criticising yourself. Like everything we have described in this book, it's not your fault that you have ended up with self-critical thoughts; these will have developed over time for a whole host of reasons particular to you and your life. If you are in a hole, stop digging, and start working out how to climb out. Actively working on your sense of esteem will benefit you in all areas of your life. If this exercise is too difficult to do, try using other self-help resources specifically focused on low self-esteem found in the resources section of this book.

To Sum Up

- Every parent worries from time to time
- For some mums, worry can become a significant and distressing problem

- Worry becomes a problem when you find it difficult to stop repetitively thinking about things going wrong in the future
- You can work on reducing your worries by recognising when you are 'catastrophising' and by practising shifting your focus of attention away from worries
- You can test out your ideas or beliefs about worrying – for example that worry helps you to be prepared, or be in control, or have total certainty
- You can learn to recognise the worries you can effectively problem solve and let go of the worry you can't
- You can work on spotting and reducing self-critical thinking which can make worry worse

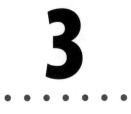

Unwanted Intrusive Thoughts of Harm (Obsessive Compulsive Disorder)

In this chapter you will learn:

➤ What intrusive thoughts are and why everyone has them

➤ Why new parents may get more of these thoughts

➤ How our interpretations and responses to the thoughts can make them feel worse

➤ How to respond differently to these thoughts and feel better

---

What Are Intrusive Thoughts?

So, what exactly are intrusive thoughts? We will use the term thoughts to include images, words and urges. The fact is that intrusive thoughts are the same as all our other thoughts, but these ones catch our attention and seem particularly important, often because they are about something that we strongly *do not want* to happen. A whole range of thoughts are going through our minds all the time without us particularly noticing or analysing them. Some are positive ('I'm looking forward to my holiday'), some negative ('What if I fail my exam?'), and some neutral ('I need to book my optician appointment'). It is important to remember we don't control or choose which thoughts are there, they just seem to come and go. It's part of what makes us human. We have a unique ability to hold things in mind which are not actually happening and sometimes don't even exist (unicorns?). Our creativity and ability to imagine and plan depend on it. It would be a strange existence if we had to plan our thoughts and could only think what we had already thought.

Thoughts pop up in our minds all the time, but usually they are not *completely* random. In many instances they are linked to things that are going on in our life and the situation we are in. Often thoughts of something negative happening will occur when there is an element of uncertainty, unfamiliarity and importantly a sense of agency, or responsibility. By agency, we mean our sense that there is something that we could do or not do in the situation that would influence the outcome. For example, the thought 'I could easily jump' will have a particular resonance if it pops into our mind when we are standing at the top of a cliff rather than the bottom.

It is also at these times that such thoughts might stand out and we give them more attention than we might at other times. An image of jumping off the cliff might flash into our mind with a small hit of adrenalin and cause us to take a step backwards, even though we would never jump, or even stand close to the edge. The context is therefore really important to the type of thoughts that are there, how they make you feel, and what you do about them.

Let's now consider the type of thoughts that are really common to have during pregnancy or after having a baby.

> *'Image of stabbing the baby'*
> *'I've eaten something that could harm the baby'*
> *'What if I sexually abused her?'*

'What if I drop him?'
'Urge to puncture the fontanelle'

Would it surprise you to learn that these are examples of intrusive thoughts experienced by parents who did *not* have anxiety or any other kind of psychological problem? That's right – an important research study which surveyed parents in the months after birth found that *all* parents have occasional upsetting thoughts of accidentally harming their baby, and at least half reported unwanted thoughts of deliberate harm. This last figure is possibly an underestimate (it is likely that some people would not have reported their worst intrusive thoughts), but nonetheless the survey was an important step in establishing that having occasional intrusive thoughts of all kinds is a *normal experience* for parents [1].

The researchers found that a whole range of horrible thoughts occurred to at least some parents in the group, including those of violent harm and sexual abuse. An important point to note here is that there was no risk of harming their baby due to these thoughts. Over the past thirty years or so, a whole host of studies have been conducted about intrusive thoughts in the general (non-pregnant / postnatal) population which also found that all sorts of intrusive thoughts of violence, sex, death and other inappropriateness occur to people very frequently, without any evidence that people act on such thoughts. This makes sense if you remember that the thoughts flash up as examples of things we want to avoid happening. This was the first study to look exclusively at postnatal women and further studies have replicated this finding with mothers and fathers, finding that such thoughts are common in both parents.

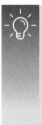 **KEY IDEA**

Horrible intrusive thoughts are common and do not mean that you want to, or will, act on them. Upsetting thoughts about your pregnancy or newborn baby are very unpleasant to experience, but do not mean that you are bad or dangerous – it is actually normal to have these thoughts.

Why Do Parents Get Unwanted Intrusive Thoughts?

If you are pregnant or if you have recently had a baby, thoughts about harm coming to your child are very likely to occur. These differ from the 'what if' type of worries we address in Chapters 2 and 8 (excessive worrying and pregnancy-related anxiety). The thoughts we are considering in this chapter are thoughts and images of something bad happening due to our own actions or inactions, that can also make us worry about why the thoughts are there in the first place. The situation of having a baby has all the qualities that would make you *notice* these thoughts: the topic of the thoughts is something important to you (a baby!), there is an element of uncertainty about their safety (they are vulnerable), and of course as a parent, you are in a very direct way responsible for keeping them safe.

Unwanted intrusive thoughts occur throughout pregnancy and seem to peak in intensity at around three months after birth [2]. They occur to both mothers and fathers, with mothers experiencing more frequent and more distressing thoughts, possibly due to there being more emphasis on the maternal caregiving role in pregnancy and the early postnatal months. Researchers have suggested that unwanted intrusive thoughts have an evolutionary function; that is that they occur to all parents as part of a general mechanism that has evolved in response to the responsibility of looking after a baby. However, whilst it is a good idea to be alert to dangers and aware of threat to an extent when caring for a new baby, intrusive thoughts start to be a problem when we pay a great deal of attention to them and treat them as more important and significant than the situation deserves. If this happens, they stick out and stick around a lot more.

Why Can't I Get These Thoughts Out of My Head?

It's not surprising that parents get more baby-related intrusive thoughts of harm than non-parents, and these thoughts bother them more than other intrusive thoughts of harm which seem less relevant [3]. When they occur, intrusive thoughts are unwanted and even mildly distressing for almost all parents – no one particularly likes thoughts of something awful happening. Some parents will even push them out of their minds or distract themselves. For most people they are a fleeting experience; the thoughts pop in and then out again and it's possible to move on and think about something else.

However, for some parents, these thoughts are experienced as very troubling, are more frequent and harder to dismiss. You may be reading this section of the book because you have unwanted intrusive thoughts that you find disturbing and are struggling to make sense of. You are certainly not alone in this. It is the case for a significant minority of parents – the latest research indicates that almost 3% of pregnant women and about 7% of postnatal women experience a level of interference from intrusive thoughts and reactions to these thoughts, that could be classified as a mental health problem. This was higher than previous figures because the researchers took care to ask not only about intrusive thoughts that anyone might have, but also about the particular ones that parents of young babies often experience [4].

So, given that the thoughts themselves are normal and occur to almost all parents, the puzzle is what makes this a problem for some and not others? The answer is in how the thoughts are interpreted and responded to. If it feels like your thoughts are signalling danger and it feels that this is not just a possibility, but that it is very likely, then to ignore them can feel very irresponsible.

For example, we know images of dropping the baby are common and most people ignore them, not interpreting them as personally significant. But if another parent has this image and thinks 'This thought means I could kill my baby and I am a terrible mother', then the thought is going to feel very different and lead to very different responses. It's a bit like an iceberg, with lots going on underneath the thoughts which appear at the top level.

 KEY IDEA

It's not the thoughts themselves that are the problem, it is what you believe the thought means that is most important.

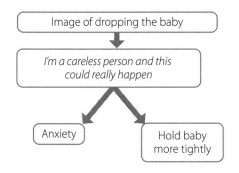

As we will discuss in detail, what you think about these thoughts, that is, this *interpretation* of the thoughts, combined with the features of the perinatal period such as sleep deprivation, feelings of responsibility, high standards and lots of other factors, leads to responding to unwanted intrusive thoughts in ways (to try to get rid of them) that can actually make them more persistent. In this way, the solution actually becomes part of the problem.

What Is the Link between Intrusive Thoughts and Obsessive Compulsive Disorder?

A key fact underpinning our understanding is that the experience of distressing and unwanted intrusive thoughts occurs on a spectrum. Almost everyone has occasional intrusive thoughts (termed 'obsessions' in obsessive compulsive disorder (OCD)) which they may try to get out of their heads using various strategies such as distraction, avoiding things, handwashing, cancelling out the thought with another word or image, and seeking reassurance (termed 'compulsions' in OCD).

However, for some people, because the thoughts feel very important and credible, they take repeated, time-consuming actions to avoid harm. If you feel low or anxious, these thoughts may also become more common and seem even more believable. When these thoughts and behaviours start to interfere and cause significant distress, taking up at least an hour a day, they would fit with a diagnosis of OCD.

OCD is the experience of repeated intrusive thoughts that bring an awareness of danger (obsessions) that are hard to dismiss, and the experience of actions aimed at reducing a sense of threat (compulsions). Whilst many people have heard about OCD related to fears of contamination and washing, which are common forms of OCD in the perinatal period, OCD about intrusive thoughts of accidental harm or deliberate harm is much less talked about and less well known, although it is possibly even *more* common at this time.

There is now good evidence that pregnancy and the postnatal period in particular is a time of increased risk for OCD – in the general population about 1–2% of people will have OCD at any one time. Several studies have shown rates of about double this in perinatal women and, as detailed above, rates may be up to 7% in the postnatal period when women are asked about specific baby-related intrusive thoughts.

'Perinatal OCD' or 'maternal OCD' as it has become known (although it also happens to fathers) is OCD that occurs during pregnancy or the postnatal period. It is often about aspects of looking after the baby, but it can be about other unrelated areas of life too. OCD often moves from theme to theme in a person's life, as it tends to focus on what is meaningful and important to them at the time, so it is not uncommon for people to have had intrusive thoughts about other things in the past to develop new concerns related to pregnancy and taking care of the baby. For many, this may not have reached the level of interference that constitutes a diagnosable mental health problem, but it is the same thinking style that comes into play.

So, wherever you might be on this spectrum from occasional upset and interference from intrusive thoughts, through to a more severe and distressing experience, understanding how OCD thinking works and how it can start to dictate your behaviour can be very helpful in preventing it interfering now and in the future.

Intrusive Thoughts in Pregnancy

Anthea

A few months after an early miscarriage, Anthea was very happy to be pregnant again and wanted to give everything the best chance of success. However, as things went on, she was becoming increasingly worried about harm coming to the baby. Always a very careful person, Anthea began to worry obsessively about the food she ate, the ingredients in it, and who might have touched it in the food preparation process.

By the time she was 20 weeks pregnant, she washed her hands not only every time she touched food, but when she was in contact with something which could touch her food, such as plates and cutlery. She stopped eating food that she had not prepared herself, but soon became concerned about food bought from the supermarket. Even though she knew she should eat fresh fruit and vegetables, she could not rule out the possibility that something had contaminated her food.

Anthea started to worry about wider forms of contamination, carefully checking skin creams and bath products for signs of ingredients that could potentially cause harm to her baby. She spent many hours on the Internet reading the latest research evidence on harm to the unborn fetus, and frequently asked her partner for reassurance that things were safe, before double checking on the Internet later. Anthea started to find it difficult to go to unfamiliar places, and soon to go out much at all.

Postnatal Intrusive Thoughts of Harm

Maya

Maya had experienced a relatively uncomplicated first pregnancy and was very much looking forward to meeting her baby son Heston. However, the birth was not exactly the calm hypnobirthing experience she had dreamed of, and Heston was eventually born after 18 hours of labour by ventouse delivery.

Glad to be over it, Maya clearly recalled the moment that Heston was finally handed to her and the sense of relief she felt. However, just after this, as she looked down at him, an image of strangling Heston intruded into Maya's mind. It was so intense that it felt like an almost physical urge. Feeling terrified and ashamed of what was in her mind, she felt completely unable to tell anyone, and pushed the thought away. Maya kept up a brave face, but was terrified that the thoughts had unlocked some terrible truth about herself in which her true evil nature would take control. In the early days she made sure to be with her husband Barry at all times and could barely sleep due to anxiety about the thought that was now recurring in her mind. She wondered how she was going to cope with being alone with Heston.

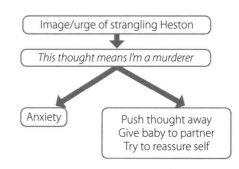

Anthea and Maya were both experiencing intrusive thoughts that they felt they couldn't ignore. For them, the thoughts seemed meaningful and were signalling that their babies were at risk, and therefore to ignore them would have been dangerous and irresponsible. It is this *interpretation* or belief that explains why the thoughts seemed so important and led them to act to try and prevent harm – in ways that made sense given what they believed. The last thing they wanted was for their baby to be harmed.

Specific intrusive thoughts can be about almost anything. As detailed above, common thoughts related to *accidentally* harming the baby include dropping them, running the bath water too hot, leaving them somewhere, the baby choking, holding them incorrectly, smothering them accidentally. Common thoughts of *deliberate* harm include touching their genitals, stabbing them, drowning them, or screaming at them. Have a look at the checklist below to see several examples of common perinatal intrusive thoughts and common responses.

Checklist of common baby-specific thoughts

Pregnancy baby-related intrusive thoughts
I've eaten something which can harm the baby
I may have been exposed to a toxin (animal faeces etc.)
My phone is giving off radiation
The baby is not my partner's (I slept with someone without knowing it)
I might harm my baby on purpose
Postnatal baby-related intrusive thoughts
I could accidentally suffocate the baby
I could drop the baby
Sexual thoughts about the baby
The baby may get ill from contamination
The baby may die from SIDS (cot death)
The baby could have an accident if I'm not careful enough
I could harm the baby intentionally (e.g. strangling, smothering, stabbing, drowning)
I might leave the baby somewhere
The baby may contract an illness
The environment may contaminate the baby (asbestos, radiation etc.)
Does the baby have the 'right' name?
Magical thinking about bad things happening to the baby
I'm not completely certain I love the baby?
I've made a mistake becoming a parent?
The baby will be psychologically damaged from me shouting at them?
If someone I don't like holds the baby, they will be contaminated by them

Responses to intrusive thoughts
Reassure myself
Seek reassurance from others (partner, family, professional)
Checking (the baby, the Internet, the surroundings)
Avoidance (situations, people, things, states)
Washing / cleaning
Pushing thoughts away / replacing a 'bad' thought with a good one
Mental distraction (trying to think about something else)
Religion / prayer
Behavioural distraction (trying to do something else)
Criticise myself for having horrible thoughts or not being good enough
Perform a ritual (counting, tapping, straightening)

It's important to remember that this could never be an exhaustive list – if your particular thought, image or sensation is not mentioned, that does not mean it's therefore weird or sinister. Intrusive thoughts could be about *anything* and it would be impossible to list them all.

Sometimes parents have unwanted intrusive thoughts which are not directly related to the baby at all, although they are still bothered by what the thought seems to mean about them, and this can in turn make them feel like they are less competent or worthy as parents and as people. For example, images of making a mistake, or a blasphemous thought, or accidentally leaving the stove on. The key thing to work out now is what your thought seems to mean to you, or what you think it means about you that the thought is in your mind. The themes that people find troubling are usually around the idea of doing something bad or wrong now or in the future, or having done something like this in the past and not realised. Often this then boils down to an idea that you are, or could be, a bad person, that you may somehow be 'crazy' and could lose control, or that you are fundamentally incompetent. So 'mad, bad or dangerous to know'.

Working Out the Meaning of Intrusive Thoughts

Sometimes people will say that afterwards they feel less convinced by their thoughts than they do in the moment. In order to access the interpretation, it's important to dig down into the meaning of your thoughts *at the time*. Try to think of a particular time when you were bothered by an intrusive thought, then freeze frame at the moment the thought struck. See how this works for Anthea and Maya:

Anthea

What thoughts are bothering you?	My food is contaminated with something that will harm the baby What if there is something toxic in the environment that will harm the baby?
What's so bad about having this thought?	I don't want any harm to come to the baby
What makes it hard to ignore or dismiss?	Now I've had this thought, it feels important and that it would be irresponsible to dismiss it
What does the fact you are having these thoughts mean about you?	I must do absolutely everything to eliminate all risk to my unborn baby
What's the worst thing about this thought?	I'm a careless and negligent mother unless I am absolutely certain that I am not harming my baby
And what's the very worst thing about this?	My baby will be born with serious irreversible health problems and it will be my fault

Maya

What thoughts are bothering you?	Strangling my baby
What's so bad about having this thought?	No decent mother would have this thought
What makes it hard to ignore or dismiss?	I should only experience love for my baby
What does the fact you are having these thoughts mean about you?	Having this thought means I must be a horrible person
What's the worst thing about this thought?	Having this thought is as bad as actually harming my baby
And what's the very worst thing about this?	I am a terrible person

Once you have worked out what the thoughts seem to mean, it may make more sense of why they are so hard to dismiss. For Anthea and Maya, it was about something very personally important and significant. For you, it may be linked to beliefs you have held about yourself for a long time – for example you may have always thought you were odd, or you might have always lacked confidence in yourself, or it may be linked to ideas about how the world works that have not been a problem until now. For example, Anthea felt that she was someone who often made mistakes, remembering a time as a child she ran a bath and forgot about it, leading to some fairly negative consequences for the bathroom. Although non-practising now, Maya had been brought up in a religion which emphasised that you could sin by merely thinking something bad.

Decades of research in OCD has helped identify some particular beliefs that are relevant to the experience of intrusive thoughts. Here are some common ones:

- Thoughts are facts
- Thinking things is the same as doing them on a moral level
- Thinking something makes it more likely to happen
- Not preventing harm is the same as causing harm
- Any influence is the same as total responsibility – if it's possible I can prevent something bad, I must do everything I can
- I must do everything perfectly

Anthea believed that she was 100% responsible for eliminating all risk. Maya believed that thinking something bad was the same as doing it. You may notice that these beliefs and rules sound quite extreme and inflexible, which is usually a clue that they aren't very helpful. The context in which you experience the thought is really important. The idea that you didn't try hard enough to prevent something bad happening may not feel quite as crucial in other situations, like when at work or socialising with friends. But it feels *really* important when you are pregnant or a parent, when the main task *is* taking care of and being responsible for a small vulnerable person. It is these underlying beliefs that are crucial to understanding what is different between those people who are very bothered by intrusive thoughts compared to those who are not.

If you are distressed by intrusive thoughts, even if you haven't put them into words before, it is very likely that some version of these beliefs is part of your thinking. We will discuss where beliefs might come from later in this chapter.

OVER TO YOU

What Are My Intrusive Thoughts and Why Do They Bother Me So Much?

You could list your thoughts in the following table or use the previous checklist to work out how your own thoughts follow this pattern. If it feels too hard to write down the full thought, just jot a word or two so that you know what you are referring to. The important thing at this point is to try and understand what you think the thoughts mean, or what they say about you. If this meaning is not obvious at first, one way to find out is to ask yourself, 'What is the worst thing about that?' or 'What do I ultimately fear will happen if I ignore this thought?'.

You can use the questions below to help you work out what your thoughts mean to you.

What thoughts are bothering you?
What's so bad about having these thoughts?
What makes them hard to ignore or dismiss?
What does the fact you are having these thoughts mean about you?
What's the worst thing about these thoughts?
What's the very worst thing about this situation?

When the belief is active in your thinking, it leads to particular physical or mental responses that make perfect sense, *given the meaning that is activated*. However, it is these reactions that also become part of the problem, as they can, in a number of ways, make the belief seem more credible, and the thoughts more important. Read on to understand why.

What Makes the Thoughts So Hard to Dismiss: Things in the Present

Anxiety and Low Mood

You have probably reflected at times that your thoughts and the meaning you attach to them might not be completely accurate, or that your behaviour is excessive, but it's very hard to remember this when you are feeling anxious and under threat.

This is due to the nature of anxiety itself. Let's consider what anxiety is and what it does, and how this might explain this difference. If you have a thought that you find scary, this sends a shot of adrenaline through your brain and body that activates your 'threat system' and sends a whole range of biological processes into action. You may have heard of the 'fight or flight' mechanism that prepares us for action in the face of threat. As well as increasing heart rate in order to allow us to move fast, another effect of this is a narrowing of focus in our minds (see Chapter 1 for further information). The biological system that deals with threat affects how and what we think, as well as what we do. If a tiger is running towards us, it wouldn't be helpful if we were easily distracted by something else, so in order to keep us safe, our threat system can activate even when the 'threat' is not as obvious as a predator. The system is set up to be triggered by potential or ambiguous threat – better to think you saw a tiger that wasn't there nine times out of ten than get eaten. So, as well as anxiety being caused by the thought in the first place, the *feeling* of anxiety can itself make us *believe* that a threat is more real.

> When Anthea was about to eat a tin of sardines for lunch, she immediately had the doubt 'What if this is contaminated with other fish that are toxic in pregnancy?'. She felt very anxious at the thought of threat to her unborn baby, and the idea kicked in that she had to be completely certain about the safety of the food, otherwise she was a bad and irresponsible mother capable of harming

her baby. She felt sick, her heart raced and her hands shook as she handled the tin. These feelings made her more convinced that there was something to worry about, and that this was a real threat that she must deal with.

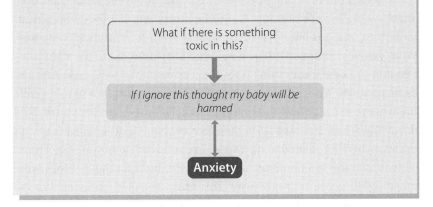

This is tricky, as it sets up a 'vicious circle' – the belief about the intrusive thought causes anxiety, and the feeling of anxiety makes the belief seem more convincing. When anxiety subsides, it is often easier to see that this may not be completely right, or acknowledge that it might be excessive. Unfortunately, we can't just dial down anxiety directly, but it's important to be aware of how mood influences what we experience. Sometimes we feel that there must be something to be afraid of just because we feel anxious, in a process called 'emotional reasoning'. However, the flaw in this is that the emotion is caused by what we fear rather than by actual danger.

Other emotions that might be present, such as depression and disgust, can also work in the same way, seeming to confirm our negative thoughts and beliefs. Emotions have a powerful effect on how we feel and how we think. It is often the case that there is a lot going on in people's lives during pregnancy and the postnatal period, in terms of worries and stress to do with romantic and family relationships, financial worries, housing and just the sheer relentless demand of it all. All these factors have an indirect effect by raising general levels of anxiety and depression that in turn mean specific anxiety about the meaning of intrusive thoughts is more easily triggered.

What We Pay Attention To

Once we notice and flag something as a threat, we tend to notice more of it and pick it out of all the possible things that could catch our attention. There are thousands of things in our environment that we could pay attention to, and our brains have to process this information in some way. What catches our focus is based on what is meaningful to us, without us needing to consciously think about it. For example, when you first became pregnant, you might have seen with new eyes just how many people there are pushing prams and holding children by the hand as you walked down the street. Perhaps it seemed like everyone had a baby! It wasn't because there happened to be a spike in the birth rate in your exact postcode at just the moment you were pregnant, but that these things were meaningful to you in a new way. This effect is called 'salience'. We are particularly efficient at noticing things which fit with our sense of threat. If there was suddenly a newsflash about a form of contagious scurvy that was passed on by pigeons, what do you think you would notice when you went outside?

So, if a thought seems to be dangerous, what will your mind be filtering and noticing? For Anthea, this meant noticing an increasing number of things which seemed like a source of contamination, with the net being cast wider and wider as time went on. The more she thought about it, the less safe she felt. For Maya, it was paying increasing attention to her thoughts, and then having the sense they were coming at her at all times. Attention is usually an automatic process, so we may not be aware of it at work. Maya interpreted the fact she was having lots of thoughts as further evidence that the thoughts were dangerous and that she really was a bad person. You may have spotted that this is another vicious circle – the more thoughts we notice, the more we have.

We can also 'selectively attend' to things in our past that fit with the scary belief rather than think of all the hundreds or thousands of times that it hasn't happened. For example, Anthea could recall reading a news story

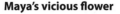

Maya's vicious flower

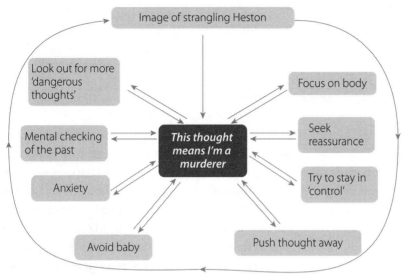

about severe illness in a pregnant mother caused by food poisoning, but did not recall information about how many pregnant women *do not* get food poisoning.

This can also happen with physical sensations. This is particularly common if people have intrusive thoughts of sexual or violent harm who might check in with themselves to ensure they are not actually physically aroused. This can go wrong; trying to work out if there are signs you are aroused is complicated if you are anxious and there is a lot of blood pumping around your body. We can illustrate with an exercise: if you take a few moments to *really* concentrate and focus your attention on the soles of your feet right now, you may be able to feel your shoes or socks if you are wearing them, or the ground underneath your feet. Perhaps you can even feel the individual toes. Were you noticing all these things a moment ago? This is a good example of how attention is like a zoom lens, amplifying what is there and even bringing on new sensations. If you have had this experience and interpreted it as 'evidence' that you want to act on thoughts, it can be very disturbing.

KEY IDEA

We notice things that fit with our frightening ideas – our attention is drawn towards 'evidence' that something bad could or has happened.

Pushing Thoughts Away

If you experience unpleasant thoughts or images of bad things happening to your baby, it may seem like the only thing you can do is to try and block them out of your mind or try and distract yourself. However, pushing thoughts away can actually increase the frequency of thoughts and add to their significance. If you tried really hard right now to think of anything at all, *apart* from a pink elephant, so definitely not its big pink trunk and huge tusks, you might find that it is quite difficult to eliminate this image completely from your mind now. In order not to think of something, you have to have an idea of what it is you don't want to think about and before you know it ... the idea is in your mind. Furthermore, in pushing the thought away, you are treating it as unacceptable and dangerous, and something that needs a response. This behaviour makes sense, given you have interpreted the thoughts as dangerous, but drags attention back towards the thoughts. You might experience what is known in psychology as the 'rebound effect' – that pushing a thought away can cause you to have more thoughts. You might have spotted that this is another vicious circle, as the more thoughts you have, the more believable becomes the idea that you are in danger. This was certainly the case for Maya, who believed that having the thoughts in the first place meant she was a bad mother. As a result, she desperately tried not to have these thoughts, and to get the images out of her mind, which had the counterproductive effect of producing more thoughts, which further strengthened her belief in her 'badness'.

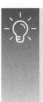

KEY IDEA

Trying not to think about something makes you think about it more, and reinforces the idea that the thought means something bad or dangerous.

Things You Do to Try and Stay Safe (Safety-seeking Behaviours)

If you feel there is a danger that you can prevent, then it makes sense to try and do something about it. We call these behaviours 'safety-seeking behaviours.' For Anthea it was careful researching of ingredients and lots of hand-washing and cleaning. When women become pregnant, there is a lot of guidance regarding things to do and things to avoid. Generally, this is helpful and pregnant women are more aware than they were before of what they are ingesting and the need for good hygiene. However, you may have heard the messages about potential problems as a signal that you and your baby are very vulnerable to specific or multiple threats. Women are given a clear message that it is their job to follow the guidance to keep their baby safe, but unfortunately the 'rules' can be less clear and are often being updated with new information. This can cause considerable anxiety about the outcome of the pregnancy (see Chapter 8 on pregnancy-related anxiety), and it can also feel like the onus is on you to do as much as possible to avoid all types of harm.

For women like Anthea experiencing anxiety, it is very hard to know when to stop. The more she sought clarification by researching on the Internet, the less sure she felt about what precautions were enough. It was rare for her to find statements saying that a certain ingredient was 100% safe for pregnant women, even things she had previously assumed were fine and knew that several of her friends used. Once she realised that there was some doubt, she found it very hard to continue eating or using the product. She told herself that it would be her fault if something happened to the baby as it could have been avoided. At each antenatal check she had, Anthea felt that things were only going alright because she was doing so much to stay safe. This was only until the next thought or doubt occurred.

Maya was so afraid that she might act on her thoughts of harming Heston that she tried to make sure people were with her all the time and held him by not touching his neck if she could. She would put him down at every opportunity, and if this was not possible, she would try to keep her hands in a stiff position and monitor them constantly. Maya took a whole range of other measures to try and prevent herself from losing control. She thought that if she avoided coffee, she would be 'safer' around him, and even tried to avoid sleep deprivation for the same reason (an impossible task with a newborn!). By doing all these things, Maya was buying into the idea that the reason she had not acted on her thoughts was because of her precautions. However, she never felt very safe, and believed she could never 'let her guard down'.

The Logic of 'It Hasn't Happened So It Must Be Working'

A man was travelling between Birmingham and Manchester by train, taking tissues out of his pocket and throwing them out of the window, one at a time. The ticket inspectors, intrigued by his behaviour, asked what on earth he was doing. 'I'm keeping elephants off the track', the man replied. 'What?!' they said. 'There aren't any elephants here.' 'Exactly!' he said.

KEY IDEA

Safety-seeking behaviours can take a variety of forms, from checking, seeking reassurance, avoidance and many others. Taking excessive precautions to try to feel safer increases anxiety. You miss out on the opportunity to find out what would happen if you didn't take these precautions.

Avoidance

One way we have of trying to manage danger is avoiding it altogether. You can see how Anthea started to avoid certain foods and places. Maya avoided being alone with her baby as much as she could. This was understandable given their fears, but there were important unintended consequences – they missed out on nice experiences, continued to feel anxious and had frequent disagreements with their partners about what was going on. Even though she was doing it for reasons that made sense given her fears, Maya felt like a bad mum for avoiding her baby, which put her in a lose-lose situation. For both Anthea and Maya, they thought that everything they were doing to manage danger was necessary and the reason they believed this was that nothing bad had happened. Unfortunately, what they did not know was that this would have been the case anyway. Avoidance stops you finding this out.

KEY IDEA

Avoidance stops you finding out how the world really is.

Seeking Reassurance and Trying to be Certain

It is natural to seek reassurance when we feel uncertain about something. Anthea was seeking reassurance repeatedly from her partner about whether things were safe in pregnancy. Maya was not able to speak with her partner directly about her thoughts, but repeatedly sought reassurance about whether she was a good mum in other ways, from her partner and loved ones, and by comparing herself with other mums. The problem about repetitive reassurance seeking is that it isn't reassuring. This is self-evident when you think about it – if it worked, then we wouldn't need to repeat it. The problem is that the situation feels so dangerous that the required level of certainty is set too high – Anthea and Maya were seeking complete certainty that their babies were safe. We can never be 100% certain, but this is ok. In other situations, like driving a car for example, we take sensible precautions, but we do not generally require total certainty that things will be safe before we do them. This is an impossible standard. When Anthea asked her partner if he was *completely* sure that things were safe to eat, he had to say that he couldn't be 100% sure, leading her to feel more doubt and anxiety. If any parent was to ask themselves 'How can I be *certain* I'm being a good enough parent?', they would probably start to remember all the times when they didn't act perfectly. Checking generally works in the same way, in that we are trying so hard to be certain that we actually increase the focus on the small level of doubt that remains.

KEY IDEA

Trying to be completely certain increases doubt and anxiety.

Things You Do in Your Head

Intrusive thoughts that bother us can trigger a process of internal dialogue which can take a number of forms, all of which have the same effect of keeping anxiety going.

Mental Checking of Past Experiences

Maya would go over incidents in her life to work out if there were any clues as to her 'real' nature, spending hours thinking if she had done anything bad in the past and what it meant. She also pondered if she was a bad parent in other ways (e.g. I once had a sexual thought about a colleague which means I'm untrustworthy).

> She would carefully read news stories about mothers who had harmed their children in order to work out if she was similar, and to try to get inside their heads to work out what thoughts might have led them to harm. She noted that, like her, they were low and alone with their children, not thinking about the millions of other women in this situation that do not harm anyone. By raking over ambiguous information to look for certainty in this way, she only felt more doubt; these processes only served to increase her fear that she might be a danger.

Try comparing this with other experiences of intrusive thoughts. If you have ever had less troubling intrusive thoughts prior to pregnancy (e.g. 'I could push this person in front of the train when standing at a busy station'; 'I might blurt something out at a wedding ceremony'), then it's also probable that you didn't wrestle with yourself or try to be certain that the thought didn't have any deeper meaning. You didn't treat it as having any particular importance, and as a result, it probably didn't return very frequently.

Maya knew in her heart that she was not going to act on her thoughts, but was stuck in a cycle of questioning herself about *why* she was having the thoughts: 'What does it mean about me if I have these thoughts in the first place, and if I *don't* worry about being a murderer then what does *that* say about me?'. The problem was tying her up in knots.

Anthea would try and replay experiences of going to certain places in her mind to make sure that she hadn't done anything that could harm the baby. However, when she did this, she of course couldn't recall in exact detail what she had done or eaten or touched, leading to more anxiety.

Counting, Praying, Replacing Thoughts with Other Thoughts, Lucky Numbers ...

Other mental processes might be rumination about bad things happening, praying in a ritualised way, or magical responses (saying the name of everyone you love in your mind before you go to bed). All of these processes function in the same way in that they reinforce the idea that your thoughts are important and dangerous.

Self-criticism

Maya would criticise herself for having intrusive thoughts in the first place; she felt that it was important that she did not allow herself to feel better, because she was having such terrible thoughts. She believed that to do so might be allowing herself to somehow accept that the thoughts were ok, which in her view would mean that she was a bad person. This was a very unhelpful spiral and of course kept her feeling awful.

Anthea alternately criticised herself for not doing enough or for being 'silly' and doing too much. In both cases, this (unjustified and harsh) self-talk did nothing to alleviate their anxiety and certainly made them feel worse. See Chapters 2 and 6 for more on tackling self-criticism.

Sleep and Hormones

For most people, disrupted sleep is part of the territory of being pregnant and caring for an infant, and it goes without saying that being deprived of sleep has some impact on our mood. But it can also directly impact how we experience intrusive thoughts. Research has shown that sleep disruption can impact on the frequency of intrusive thoughts, and also how believable they are. Although just getting more sleep is not often straightforward, it is important to know, especially when you are in the thick of it, that sleep deprivation has an impact on intrusive thoughts and it is something that improves with time, as your opportunity to sleep more and for longer periods increases (we hope!).

Hormonal changes are an essential part of the journey through pregnancy and birth. There is ample evidence which shows that changes in hormone levels can affect mood and that some people may be more sensitive than others to changes in hormone levels. A handful of studies have examined a link between OCD symptoms and hormones, with mixed findings. Some women reported a worsening of OCD symptoms during pregnancy, while others reported an improvement, so it is difficult to make any generalisations [5]. It's another factor to consider that might be relevant for you as an individual.

Similarly, the experience of ongoing physical pain can affect our thinking in a number of ways, making us more irritable and less able to think flexibly. Unfortunately, this can occur in pregnancy and in the postnatal period. It's another indirect factor that can play a role.

Putting all these things together, there are a number of factors in the present that can make thoughts appear more believable and important by operating as simultaneous vicious circles. We call this the 'vicious flower' of understanding OCD. You can see Maya's vicious flower above and Anthea's vicious flower below:

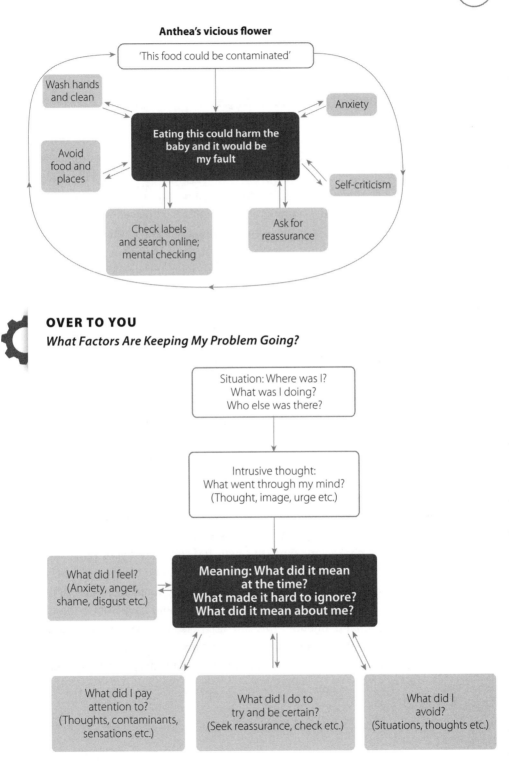

Anthea's vicious flower

'This food could be contaminated'

Wash hands and clean

Anxiety

Eating this could harm the baby and it would be my fault

Avoid food and places

Self-criticism

Check labels and search online; mental checking

Ask for reassurance

OVER TO YOU

What Factors Are Keeping My Problem Going?

Situation: Where was I?
What was I doing?
Who else was there?

Intrusive thought:
What went through my mind?
(Thought, image, urge etc.)

Meaning: What did it mean at the time?
What made it hard to ignore?
What did it mean about me?

What did I feel?
(Anxiety, anger, shame, disgust etc.)

What did I pay attention to?
(Thoughts, contaminants, sensations etc.)

What did I do to try and be certain?
(Seek reassurance, check etc.)

What did I avoid?
(Situations, thoughts etc.)

What Makes the Thoughts So Hard to Dismiss: Things in the Past

Going Through Big Life Changes

OCD often emerges during times of transition. These might be stressful events like changing school or experiencing turbulence at home from parental divorce, but it can also be seemingly positive events like leaving home or getting a new job. Transitions can be hard to navigate, leading to changes in roles, uncertainties and sometimes increased responsibilities. So even if a transition may seem like a really positive thing, aspects of it can lead OCD to emerge. Some people may have experienced OCD or that type of thinking before. However, for many women, like Maya, the onset of the problem is new in the perinatal period and is very unexpected. If this has happened, it can feel like it fits with the idea that you are vulnerable or somehow crazy. We have discussed how the new context of the perinatal period can give normal thoughts a new meaning. There is some evidence that other elements of the perinatal and maternity experience can also play a role.

Trauma and Birth-related Traumas

Traumas are difficult and impact anyone they happen to, to some extent. The experience of traumatic birth or miscarriage can for some women play a role in developing OCD (see Chapter 7 on trauma and Chapter 8 on pregnancy-related anxiety for more detailed information on how to manage these problems). It goes without saying that these kinds of traumatic experiences shake your sense of safety and sometimes your sense of self. Research tells us that quite a lot of people develop intrusive thoughts and compulsions after a trauma. In addition, unwarranted self-blame is often a feature, with people left wondering if they could have done something to prevent what happened. This can also make you overcompensate with trying to get things 'right' this time. Unfortunately, although it is not talked about enough, experiences of miscarriage, stillbirth and traumatic births are quite common. Although there is no evidence that women with OCD have suffered greater rates of these events, for some people these experiences can be particularly hard to process, and it is this that can play a role in ramping up a sense of threat in later pregnancies. It makes sense that these kinds of experiences can lead to more intrusive thoughts as your threat system kicks in.

Similarly, in vitro fertilisation (IVF) is almost always a mentally and physically challenging experience to go through. For many women it starts after a long period of difficult pregnancy experiences and loss. The process itself involves lots of questioning, lots of uncertainty (and lots of hope), but also intense physical monitoring that can emphasise risk and responsibility. For some people, the stress associated with the process can lead to or exacerbate intrusive thoughts and behaviours related to getting things exactly right, and that sense of uncertainty is there right through the pregnancy.

We have conducted research into intrusive thoughts with parents with a baby on the Neonatal Intensive Care Unit (NICU). These parents often have high levels of anxiety and can feel very traumatised by their experiences. Our study also found that they had very frequent intrusive thoughts of both accidental and deliberate harm coming to the baby. This supports the idea that these thoughts and experiences are an understandable response to the demands of stress, uncertainty and responsibility that are really acute in the NICU environment.

Background Beliefs

Beliefs are not the same as facts. We all have a set of beliefs about how the world works, even if we have never put them into words. They may come from our background culture, the way we were brought up and specific experiences, and usually from a combination of all these things. Often these beliefs cause us no trouble, until a certain experience brings particularly negative or rigid beliefs to the forefront. They can be beliefs about our role in the world such as 'I must do everything perfectly', or about how thoughts work ('I should never sin in thought or word or deed'). Sometimes we are given messages by our upbringing. Perhaps you were not given any responsibility as a child, leading you to conclude 'I am not competent', or perhaps you were given lots of responsibility (so you felt 'It is my job to look after everybody'). These kind of background ideas can be part of the explanation of why the thoughts seem so important.

Particular incidents in childhood can reinforce ideas which become problematic later, for example having the random thought 'I wish my cat would die' and then coincidentally this happening, leading to a conclusion that 'My thoughts have power.' Sometimes this is reinforced by cultural messages from religion to 'the power of positive thinking' that are taken very literally. We would argue that it is actions rather than thinking that really makes things happen. Horror films like to play on these ideas as well and can sometimes affect people for years after having seen them.

Perhaps you picked up an overall message that you are basically a good person, that it's ok to show and talk about emotions, to trust others and that the world is a safe enough and manageable place. But if you were given other more negative messages about yourself, the world and other people, then you can probably see how these might provide an opportunity for intrusive thoughts to feel significant and meaningful.

Rigid beliefs that you have to get everything right and do things perfectly are often associated with low mood and anxiety, because in any situation being perfect is just not sustainable. Being a parent is one of those situations. We talk more about developing fairer, more helpful versions of these beliefs in Chapter 9. This is something that is really important – in order to do as well as you can in this situation, you need to be fair and supportive to yourself. Berating yourself for falling short of your own standards makes it harder to improve and do well.

Magical Thinking

Magical thinking is the idea that thoughts themselves have power, or ideas that things are connected in non-logical ways. This could be that thinking something more will make it more likely to happen, or that thinking is the moral equivalent of doing it. Neither of these things are true. If I want to look like a film star, unfortunately thinking about it will not make it happen. It would take a number of (quite dramatic!) steps to actually do this. Thinking either positive or negative intrusive thoughts all day long will not make things happen – for example, you could spend all day thinking about winning the lottery, but it doesn't mean that it happens. If you consider how many times you have had a thought and how many times it has actually happened, you will see that there is not a relationship. See below for more ways to build your confidence in this.

Popular psychology and self-help books have normalised the 'power of positive thinking' and approaches that encourage people to repeat self-affirming ideas. There is nothing wrong with being positive and self-encouraging. This might make you feel better, so you actually do go for that run or ask for that promotion. But thinking alone will not make these outcomes happen.

In terms of thoughts having a moral equivalent to deeds, we discussed the evidence about what intrusive thoughts are, and how having occasional negative thoughts is a part of being human. Sometimes it is argued that those who do terrible things must have had the thought before this, but it's important to remember that they decided that it was something they *wanted* to do. Distressing intrusive thoughts are about things we do not want to happen and are not associated with risk of harm in any study.

Moving Forward: Theory A / Theory B

We have shown you how a whole range of reactions can be provoked by the meaning you give to the thoughts, and that each of those reactions can lead to this meaning seeming more powerful in the moment. Before this it may not have occurred to you to consider thoughts in other ways, so everything you have been doing makes sense given the information that was available to you up to now. However, we know that people who are less bothered by intrusions give a different interpretation to their thoughts, so it is certainly possible to have a different view. For example, someone might think 'That's a horrible thought! Must be one of those unpleasant intrusions that parents get!'.

What we will do next is consider a different way of understanding *your* thoughts and experiences and examine whether this alternative is in fact a better fit, as well as what to do to help you find out if you are not sure. Earlier, we asked you to think about the meaning you give to your thoughts. Let's call this 'Theory A', the idea that these thoughts mean something terrible about you, or that something terrible will happen, usually amplified by the idea it will be your fault and it is your responsibility. The alternative is that these thoughts are part of an anxiety problem. Let's call this 'Theory B'.

Anthea's 'Theory A' was 'I need to pay attention to every signal of danger or something will happen to the baby and it will be my fault. Maya's Theory A was 'These thoughts mean I am a terrible mother and could cause harm'.

Yes but … of Course I'm Anxious if I'm a Danger!

It's possible you might be thinking, as Anthea and Maya would, that of course they need to be doing *everything they can* to keep their babies safe. This is generally true of parents of course, but being so concentrated on avoiding harm may not be the best way to do the job they want to do – to be attentive, calm, responsive parents. In this case, the problem is not that they are in or are a danger, it's that they have become excessively anxious about this.

It's important that we define the problem as best we can so that we can work out the right way to solve it.

Theory A	Theory B
The problem is … DANGER	The problem is … ANXIETY
Anthea: 'I need to pay attention to every signal of danger or something will happen to the baby and it will be my fault.'	'I have become *excessively* afraid of harm coming to the baby.'
Maya: 'My thoughts mean I am a terrible mother and will cause harm.'	'I am afraid these thoughts mean I'm a terrible mum.'

In both cases, the problem Theory B could be defined as an anxiety problem, one of *being terrified* of bad things happening, rather than one of *actually* being in danger of these things happening. The difference between these ideas is a very important point. Theory A, the idea that you are in danger (or a source of danger) of course goes along with a lot of anxiety, but in this version of events the anxiety is very much secondary to the harm. Theory B is different. Theory B says that there is no more risk than for any similar person in this situation, but that all the efforts to avoid harm have become a problem in their own right. It is the difference between actually being in a minefield or walking through the countryside and treating a field as though it had mines in it – just in case. Doing this might make you feel nervous and would get in the way of your walk. You could say that all the efforts Anthea and Maya were making to solve what they believed was a problem of imminent danger were actually just making the anxiety problem worse.

We already have a good understanding of what makes the danger idea believable in the moment and how beliefs from the past may also play a role, but let's consider the evidence for these two theories alongside each other, thinking about what we know that might underpin each idea. To do this we need to try and be really strict about what is actually evidence, rather than focusing on the fact that the outcome would be bad.

Anthea began to think of her reasons for responding to all of her thoughts and immediately considered how awful it would be if the baby was harmed. This goes without saying, but is it the same as saying she had to do *all* the things she was doing to avoid harm? Anthea found it hard to come up with other reasons to support Theory A. She was aware that most pregnant women were not doing what she was doing. She did not have any special conditions that made her more vulnerable. This itself is evidence for Theory B. She considered further what other characteristics might fit with this being a fear problem through thinking about the behaviour and views of people she knew, and her own beliefs and experiences.

Theory A	Theory B
The problem is … DANGER	The problem is … ANXIETY
I need to pay attention to every signal of danger or something will happen to the baby and it will be my fault.	*For understandable reasons, I have become preoccupied and frightened by the idea of harm coming to my baby. My efforts to try to look out for all dangers have made me constantly worried and miserable.*
What makes me think this is true?	
It would be terrible if something bad happened to the baby. Babies are harmed by toxins. There are lots of messages that harm can come to the baby if you do the wrong thing.	Other women do not take all these precautions, even those who have complications, and their babies are generally fine. I am following all the normal guidance but have added many other precautions where the link isn't clear. I felt very traumatised by my miscarriage and feel I can't go through that again, which has made me very attuned to risk. I am quite an anxious person in general (have had general anxiety before). My partner and family think I am taking excessive precautions, and that my anxiety has got in the way of my usual clear thinking.

Similarly, Maya considered her Theories A and B.

Theory A	Theory B
The problem is … DANGER	The problem is … ANXIETY
My thoughts mean *I am* a terrible mother and will cause harm.	*I am afraid* these thoughts mean I'm a terrible mum …

Theory A	Theory B
Why do I believe this?	
I have not had thoughts like this before. The thoughts are so bad they must mean something. I have hit my brother in a fight before and have done impulsive things.	I have had other intrusive thoughts in my life, but I haven't been in the situation of being a mum before. Other mums get these thoughts on occasion. Everyone has done some imperfect or impulsive things and not everyone is a killer. Other people would say I'm a good mum and I look after Heston well. I am worried about what thoughts mean which means I must care.

Looking at the two sides, it was clear that the weight of evidence was towards Theory B.

Next Anthea thought about what she would need to do if Theory A were true, and then what she would need to do if Theory B were true.

Theory A	Theory B
The problem is … DANGER	The problem is … ANXIETY
I need to pay attention to every signal of danger or something will happen to the baby and it will be my fault.	*I have become terrified of harm coming to the baby*
What do I do if I follow this idea?	
Check everything I eat; research on the Internet; ask for reassurance from partner, midwives, doctors, manufacturers; keep up with the latest research; avoid eating all food I have not made myself; don't go out.	Remember I am doing way more than normal or necessary. Follow the normal guidance. Don't research everything. Don't repeatedly ask for reassurance or delay for an hour to see if I still need it. Do things I enjoy – try to tackle things I have been avoiding. Try to be kind to myself about my anxiety.

Theory A	Theory B
What happens if I carry on doing these things?	
Very stressful and limiting. Means I can't do a lot of things I enjoy. Puts strain on my relationship. It is quite unhealthy to only eat a small range of foods and be so stressed all the time. Worried I will be like this as a parent and will be very anxious about my baby.	I will hopefully feel less anxious and preoccupied. I should have more time for other things and be able to look after myself better. Things will be better with family. I will probably be better able to manage postnatally if I can get a handle on this now.

For Anthea, a difficulty in her Theory A was that there was no real limit to what she could think of, as everything has the potential to be dangerous. This left her constantly afraid of failing and doing the wrong thing as she could barely keep up with the problem.

It is therefore really important to think about what the problem is making you do, what this is costing you, what it is stopping you doing and the problems it is causing. Intrusive thoughts and anxiety can make you feel very bad about yourself, because you can never do enough, and you feel like you are at risk of failing at every turn. They can get in the way of enjoying motherhood. A helpful way to think about Theory A is a problem of *competence* – the thoughts are saying you could muck up at any point. The alternative is that it's a problem of *confidence* – the thoughts have made you lose trust in your own judgement. This is something you can get back by taking some practical steps as we outline here.

'Better Safe than Sorry': How This Idea Keeps Anxiety Going

Anxiety had managed to convince Anthea that the more cautious she was, the safer she was. We have all heard the phrase 'better safe than sorry' and of course it can seem on the surface like a sensible idea, especially where the welfare of a baby is concerned. However, to be clear, where intrusive thoughts are in control, you are not choosing between these things. Even though she took a huge number of precautions, Anthea was really no safer than the average pregnant woman, but she was certainly feeling very sorry with the huge impact of all the things she was doing. She was trading off her current state of mind against a hypothetical threat. The level of stress and tension she was experiencing was definitely causing damage in the here and now.

The idea of an insurance policy can be another useful metaphor to understand how anxiety works. Imagine if you were offered a really comprehensive insurance policy that covered everything for your house, even as far as extensive cover for floods, earthquakes, alien invasions. You might think it sounds attractive, but what if the cost was £1 million per year? You probably wouldn't go for it. That is why it is important to consider the real costs of following the problem (Theory A), which always demands a high and often rising price for the idea of safety. Yet there is no evidence that doing these things really do make you safer, or they would be in the standard guidance.

Although Maya had different types of thoughts, the impact was similar. All her precautions and monitoring were getting in the way of enjoying her time as a mum, and left her with the distressing idea that she was a threat to her baby. The problem pushed her into a corner, in that the harder she tried to be safe, the worse she felt. This is what is so difficult when intrusive thoughts take hold.

Theory A	Theory B
The problem is … DANGER	The problem is … ANXIETY
My thoughts mean I am a terrible mother and will cause harm.	I am afraid these thoughts mean I'm a terrible mum.
What do I do if I follow this idea?	
Monitor my thoughts. Tell myself I won't act on the thoughts. Try and make sure by being very careful. Make sure I will not harm Heston.	Treat thoughts as thoughts – stop changing my behaviour when I get a thought. Don't avoid or take any extra precautions. Do all the tasks of caring for Heston whether other people are there or not. Stop pushing the thoughts away; don't try to work them out and question myself. Think the thoughts on purpose to take the power away from them. Remember that the thoughts don't mean anything about me or what I want. Trust myself more.

Theory A	Theory B
What happens if I carry on doing these things?	
It's very stressful; I feel like a terrible person; I should probably not be caring for Heston.	I should feel more confident about myself. I will feel happier. The thoughts should get less intense.

The really good news is that there is an alternative way of understanding what you are experiencing (Theory B), and that this is in all likelihood a better fit with the actual evidence of how the world really works, and who you really are. You don't have to fully believe it yet, and part of the process now is trying things out to work out which is the best approach. You may notice from reading the tables above that the way to solve an anxiety problem is almost the opposite of what you would do to deal with a problem of danger. Understanding and treating your problem as one of anxiety means tackling all the things that increase anxiety and belief in danger that we outlined earlier. These are generally all the things that go with Theory A – all the avoidance, checking, washing, cancelling out thoughts. Moving forward means approaching rather than avoiding, dropping excessive precautions, and treating yourself with self-compassion for having this problem by encouraging yourself to apply this new understanding and make changes where you can. We will discuss in more detail how to do this.

We have used common examples of contamination fears and intrusive violent thoughts to illustrate the steps for working through this type of problem. We have worked with women with all the different forms of intrusive thoughts mentioned in the checklist above, and even after many years there are still new ones that we encounter. However, the people we work with have found this framework to be helpful regardless of what the specific thoughts are, because the themes of the thoughts and the thinking patterns around problematic intrusive thoughts are very similar regardless of the content.

OVER TO YOU
My Theory B

Fill in your Theory A from the 'meaning' in your vicious flower on page 67. Try and write out your Theory B in the form shown before – 'I am afraid that …'.

Theory A	Theory B
The problem is … DANGER	The problem is … ANXIETY
My thoughts mean	
Why do I believe this?	
What do I need to do if I follow this idea?	
What happens if I carry on doing these things?	

Moving Forward: Putting Theory into Practice

Completing the Theory A / B table for yourself should help you to organise your thinking about this problem and the last two Theory B sections are essentially an action plan for what you need to do, as well as a reminder of how life will be better if you follow it. Keeping in touch with the bigger picture is very helpful in tackling anxiety. Some initial discomfort at changing things is possible, given what anxiety has been telling you about what is going on, but if you continue with the Theory B plan, this should quickly ease as you gain confidence and the new way of doing things becomes more familiar. Sometimes the phrase 'tolerating' or 'accepting uncertainty' is used: perhaps a better way of thinking about it is readjusting to a less anxious you that can manage this as well as other uncertainties.

OVER TO YOU
Reset Your Goals

Now you have a direction of travel, it's a good time to think in detail about how you want things to improve in the short- and longer term. How would you know that things were moving in the right direction? What behaviours (that you didn't do before) would you like to get rid of? What would you like to be doing that you are not doing now? Below are examples of the types of goals set by Anthea and Maya. In essence their plan was to start to do the things they had been avoiding, without the accompanying safety behaviours.

Anthea's goals	Maya's goals
Buy a tea from the local café.	Don't ask Barry to take over if anxious.
Use bath product I like (and don't check it on the Internet).	Be alone with Heston for longer periods – build up to night alone.
Wash hands less often (only before I eat, after loo, before and after food prep).	Bath Heston.
Eat out with partner Arun.	Don't seek reassurance.
Don't ask for reassurance from Arun.	Hold Heston near his neck.
Postnatal – attend a mum and baby group.	Be able to ignore thoughts.

Changing what you *do* is really important to feel better. If it feels difficult to know where to start, break down your goals into smaller steps. To help you generate your goals you could consider trying to do what the average person in a similar situation would do.

	How hard is this for me now 0 = not able to do 10 = complete success
What do I want to be doing in the next few weeks?	

What do I want to be doing in the next few months?
What do I want to be doing by this time next year?

Responding Differently to Your Intrusive Thoughts: Testing Things Out

It is hard to just respond to intrusive thoughts differently as a first step. 'Exposure' to situations that you fear is a fundamental part of treatment for anxiety as it allows you to experience these situations in a new way and find out *how the world really works*. Anxiety persuades people to avoid doing things or endure them only by taking many precautions. Putting up with some anxiety helps you find out and really accept through experience that your avoidance and precautions have been unnecessary. Part of you probably knows this – but when the anxiety kicks in you are drawn in another direction. This can lead to a gap between your head and your heart. Going purposefully into a situation without checking, washing, reassurance seeking etc., allows you to get new information and bring your head and heart together in tackling anxiety. Our term for this is 'behavioural experiment', because you are testing out your fear and finding out what happens. Remember that you have already done lots of important thinking about why it is likely to be better to do things in a Theory B way; you are not taking a 'blind risk'. You are putting the theory into practice as responding differently to your fears and intrusive thoughts is key to feeling better. It might be worth creating a note on your phone or on the fridge to remind you of why you are challenging these thoughts.

It is definitely better to plan in advance what you will do, rather than think 'The next time this comes up I would like to respond in this way.' So, for example, think *when* you will go and buy the tea from the café, what this may bring up for you and how you will tackle those thoughts and feelings. The important thing is to tune into your mental and physical safety-seeking behaviours (e.g. checking, reassurance seeking, repeating) and try to do the task without those.

When picking what to do, you may want to try activities that are directly linked to your goals or think of ones which are a stepping stone toward them at the start.

We use simple recording sheets to help plan and make sense of experiments, as writing things down can make your thoughts about the experiment and what you found out afterwards much clearer. Try and be as specific as you can in your predictions so you can compare them with what actually happened. Here are some examples of behavioural experiments.

Before the experiment		After the experiment	
Planned experiment (what / where / when)	**What is the anxious prediction (and how believable is it)?**	**What happened?**	**Does that fit better with Theory A or Theory B? Why?**
Eat dinner without washing hands first.	I will become ill (85%) and will feel very guilty (100%).	I did not become ill. I felt guilty at first but this got easier after a few hours.	B – I know this is the anxiety talking.
Using public changing facility.	Baby will become unwell tonight (50%). I will be very anxious for 2 days (90%).	Baby did develop a sniffle 3 days later, but so did my partner who was not with us – I think we got it elsewhere. I had a nice time with my friend when I was out.	B – even though the baby got ill I felt pleased that we had done something nice and I can see the sniffle wasn't to do with the outing.
Bath baby and bring on intrusive thoughts of bad things happening (rather than pushing them out of my head).	Could harm baby (80%). Will feel awful for days (100%).	I didn't harm the baby. My baby smiled and chuckled so much I was laughing myself. It was actually quite hard to keep bringing on thoughts as my mind wandered. Weirdly I felt better than usual.	B – I had not done this before, so it was a surprise.

Dealing with Feelings of Anxiety

When you first do something that you have been avoiding, you may feel a bit anxious about it. This is ok, and there is no need to avoid anxiety, as anxiety itself is not dangerous, nor a sign of impending danger related to your thoughts. When you are trying to solve an anxiety problem, the aim is to experience the anxiety and soothe yourself in ways other than avoidance or washing, checking, seeking reassurance and all the rest of it. Even if they feel like they give you some relief in the short term, it is these things that actually keep anxiety going in the longer term.

TWO KEY IDEAS:

Having a thought in your mind is not the same as it being true.
Feeling anxious is not the same as something being dangerous.

We often use the metaphor of a bully to capture what it is like to be at the mercy of your intrusive thoughts. The bully is telling you to do a whole lot of things to stay safe, even though the one thing that is actually causing harm is ... the bully. You can't really reason with a bully or just do what they want and hope things will change. You need to stand up to it. This takes courage and may make you feel a bit anxious to start with. But just like a bully, if you stand up to it you find out that it's a coward at heart with not much to say beyond 'do it or else'. You are better off without it.

Dealing with Feelings of Guilt and Excessive Responsibility

For Anthea, she knew that she needed to try and do less washing and checking. This is a scary idea, because it felt like doing any less might be dangerous and involved confronting the idea that it might be irresponsible to change. She thought about what she needed to remember in order to do it – that her problem involved trying too hard to be safe – and reminded herself that she needed to be compassionate to the fact that she had become so anxious. She didn't judge other pregnant women who did not follow her rules as irresponsible and she needed to apply this to herself. She needed to remember that her rules were not necessary and were actively unhelpful in keeping her stressed and anxious. Reminding herself of why she was doing this was useful to manage these feelings.

If you have the thought that it might be irresponsible to do things differently, it can be useful to think about all the qualities that you think are important in being a mum. You could put safety first, which is what the intrusive thoughts have been focused on. A list for a mum with a small child might include some of the following:

- Keeping him alive
- Teaching him things
- Helping him to be independent and confident
- Having fun and being playful

Now try and assign a percentage to how important each one is. You might get a pie chart at the end that looks a bit like this:

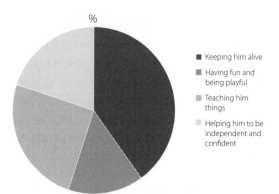

These percentages are an example and not intended as a guide – different parents have different priorities, and your list and pie chart may look very different. The point is that keeping our babies safe is only one aspect of parenting. If you were to focus on that at the expense of all others, there would be a huge cost, both to your quality of life and your baby's, and your relationship with your baby could be impacted. Anxiety would like this to happen, but remember that it's a reasonable choice to go for balance. After all, no one would get in a car to visit a loved one, or go on a plane to experience new things, if we didn't consider the full picture of risks and benefits.

Some mums feel very guilty for having intrusive thoughts of harm. Even though they know they will not act on the thoughts, and even after doing some experiments to build up confidence about this, they continue to feel that it must mean something about them. If this is the same for you, know that this feeling can take a little while to shift, but the more you treat thoughts as insignificant, the less important they seem. Remember that mulling things over in your mind is part of what keeps this problem going, and getting into this kind of 'trying to work it out' or 'cancel it out' thinking will keep the thoughts cropping up.

The idea of intrusive thoughts as an unwelcome guest at a party can be useful here. Imagine you were having a lovely time at a friend's party and someone unexpectedly turned up that you really didn't like. You can either chose to interact with them, get cross, or leave the party yourself. Or you can accept that they are there and carry on speaking to guests you do like. The first option would mean you had a miserable evening, whereas knowing they are there, but ignoring them, may give you a better chance of having a good time.

What About Situations When I Can't Know If What I Fear Has Happened, or Not For a Long Time?

Some fears are very testable, like whether or not you will act on an intrusive thought. However, many are not, such as whether the pregnancy will turn out ok, or if your child might be psychologically harmed in later life by anything that did or did not happen when they were an infant. Anxiety loves these ideas as they feed back into the 'better safe than sorry' narrative we discussed above. Remember, if you listened to all intrusive thoughts and treated them as likely rather than a tiny possibility, it would stop you from doing much at all. This would have a cost to you and your family which is a certainty, not a possibility. Keep thinking about the bigger picture and the importance of regaining your life to be able to live in the normal range, that is, in the same way as people you respect and consider are getting it right, who don't have anxiety. In our experience, when people take what *feels* like a risk to move towards this, things become much better, and the intrusive thoughts much less believable.

OVER TO YOU
Testing Things Out

What could you do tomorrow, or later this week, that helps you to over-come this problem?

Before the experiment		After the experiment	
Planned experiment (what / where / when)	What is the anxious prediction (and how believable is it)?	What happened?	Does that fit better with Theory A or B? Why?

You can use the record sheet to get going and keep a track on your progress. They can be particularly helpful over the initial weeks of testing things out, in order to keep the new framework at the front of your mind.

As time goes on you may feel more confident that you are moving from testing things out to practising your 'new normal' and getting back into day-to-day life without excessive anxiety. This is really committing to the idea that Theory B is the accurate way of understanding what is going on. You may not need the experiment sheets at this point, but do jot down the thing you are doing and take time to be pleased with yourself at every victory. It can help to revisit your goals occasionally to keep moving in the right direction.

Tackling Your Excessive Reassurance-seeking from Family and Health Professionals

When things feel uncertain it is very normal to seek reassurance. This can come in the form of seeking a more informed opinion on a topic or asking a person we trust to confirm our view when we doubt ourselves. This might be asking a midwife for reassurance about baby movements, or postnatally asking our partner if they think it's ok to give a particular food to the baby. Intrusive thoughts can often direct us to seeking reassurance about whether we are a good person, or doing the 'right' thing. Usually, reassurance is well, reassuring. We feel better, our doubts subside a bit and we move on. However, when anxiety takes hold, it is common to seek reassurance repeatedly and therefore excessively. If you find yourself asking the same question and getting the same answers, but not feeling better or more certain, your reassurance is excessive and is not working.

The reason for this is usually about what we are trying to achieve with reassurance. If we are looking for *complete* certainty that what we fear will not happen, then it is likely that whoever is providing the reassurance cannot in all honesty provide this. Seeking reassurance and checking actually makes you have more doubt, but it can also cause problems in your relationships. Putting yourself in the shoes of a person who is constantly being asked the same question (or variations on a theme), you can imagine that over time, their answers probably will become more wooden and less sincere. This is of course difficult if the person asking for reassurance is in distress.

It's important for you to share your new understanding about anxiety with the people you are asking for reassurance, preferably at a time during which you feel less anxious. Think together about what reassurance is, and what both parties can do to remind you that it is not helpful. Think about how you can work together to support you, and not help the anxiety. There is some evidence that providing support rather than reassurance at these times may be particularly effective in helping anxiety. There are no set ways to do this, and you will want to discuss together some options that both of you feel comfortable with. Here are some suggestions for alternative approaches.

Things you can do	Things your supporter can do
Label your need to ask for reassurance: 'I feel very anxious and I really want to ask you for reassurance now!'	Be encouraging; help you label it: 'This is really good, you have recognised you want reassurance.'
Try to delay seeking reassurance.	Encourage a delay: 'Shall we go for a walk for 15 minutes and see how it feels after that.'
Try to do something else instead; 'I'm feeling anxious, can I have a cuddle?'	Offer support: 'It's horrible feeling anxious. How about a hug?'

Remember seeking reassurance is a very normal thing and sometimes it is entirely appropriate. These ideas can be helpful if you find yourself in cycles of reassurance seeking which keep anxiety going. It's not the end of the world if you do ask for reassurance, but have a think afterwards about whether it was excessive and what you might do next time to reduce, delay or prevent it. You could discuss how to do this with your partner or family.

Health professionals such as midwives and doctors often provide helpful reassurance in their roles as well-informed authorities on medical issues. In fact, that is literally part of their job. They are educated and trained to provide information in answer to the questions you have and to help you think through decisions that involve weighing things up. Most aspects of medicine do not involve complete certainty, but experienced professionals can help guide you through the evidence and use their clinical experience to get the best outcomes. This is not perfect or exact. We know that sometimes professionals can be unhelpful or dismissive, or get things wrong, or be inconsistent with each other.

It can happen that, when anxiety is involved, professionals get sucked into going beyond their normal level of investigation and reassurance. Often with the best intentions, their patients are sometimes given an additional scan or procedure where not warranted as it is thought that this will provide the satisfaction and comfort that is sought. This rarely works. If, after answering your questions and doing all the routine examinations, your health professional is saying that they really don't think an extra test is necessary but that they will do it 'to put your mind at ease' then it could be a clue that this is excessive reassurance seeking. You may want to try delaying the appointment or the test, or discuss your anxiety with the professional to get their view on what is going to be most helpful. There are of course no set rules as to what is appropriate reassurance seeking, but if you notice a pattern in your own behaviour, it is worth remembering that 'more is not more' where reassurance is concerned and it is actively a part of the problem. The more you can deal with *excessive* reassurance seeking, the more useful *normal* reassurance seeking will become.

Tips For Helping a Partner Who Has Intrusive Thoughts

Anxiety can be hard on partners and loved ones. Here are some tips you can give to your partner or friends to help them help you.

1. Find out as much as you can about the problem, how it gets people stuck in doing things they know on one level aren't helpful. A shared understanding will help you help your loved one and can make it easier to empathise with how difficult it is to be stuck in the grip of upsetting intrusive thoughts.
2. Think with them about how you might best help them tackle their intrusive thoughts and responses – encouragement; a reminder of what the thoughts mean; setting goals together.
3. Talk about ways you might be able to offer encouragement and support instead of reassurance if that is a big part of what is going on.
4. Think together about setting goals that you *both* want, to reclaim life back from the problem and how you can get *fun* back into life in small or bigger ways.
5. Try and protect some time and conversation from intrusive thoughts.
6. Look after yourself and take time out where you need it, or get professional help for yourself if you think it could be of use. You can self-refer online to most talking therapies services in England, or visit your GP for a discussion. See the Resources section for further information.

Moving Forward: Beating Your Intrusive Thoughts in the Long Term

We have presented the key components to getting on top of your intrusive thoughts. These are:

- Understanding the thoughts, the meaning you attach to them and what keeps them going
- Reframing the problem as anxiety using Theory A / Theory B

- Being consistent with this in your behaviour and how you talk to yourself (being validating and kind if you feel anxious)
- Treating thoughts as thoughts
- Finding out 'how the world really works' by using behavioural experiments

Many people report that the content of their intrusive thoughts moves around, and this makes sense given that thoughts are about what is happening to us or around us at the time. It is important to be aware of this in order to be able to deal with whatever the thoughts throw at you. As you progress through pregnancy and the perinatal period, different ones may crop up, so it's good to remember that these same principles apply to whatever the topic is. A rough guide to what might influence the content of intrusive thoughts is given below.

Stage	Possible issues to navigate
Pregnancy	Adjusting to pregnancy physically – new sensations, not being able to do previously enjoyed things, sense of uncertainty. Idea of parenthood – me as a parent – will I be able to keep my child safe? Birth.
0–3 months	Issues from the birth experience – physical and mental adjustment. Issues from breastfeeding / bottle-feeding choices. Sleep deprivation. Thoughts about infant harm and vulnerability – e.g. excessive checking at night, avoidance of caregiving tasks due to unwanted intrusive thoughts of harm. The baby's name. Whether you made the wrong choice having a baby.
3–6 months	Possibly trying to get into routines – when to end co-sleeping. Feeding – breast-/bottle-feeding. Developmental milestones – are they doing what other babies are doing? Going further afield with the baby. Baby putting things in their mouth.

Stage	Possible issues to navigate
6–12 months	Sleeping. Feeding – solid feeding, choking, eating the right food. Developmental milestones – should s/he be doing this by now?
12–24+ months	Baby becoming more autonomous – exploring and more exposure to dirt and germs. Considering further pregnancies – What if I relapse?

To Sum Up

- You may be having unwanted intrusive thoughts that you find disturbing and you may struggle to make sense of them
- Unwanted intrusive thoughts of accidentally or deliberately harming the baby occur to all parents and do not mean that you intend accidental or deliberate harm, or that it is likely
- Intrusive thoughts are normal. Parents get more of these unpleasant thoughts after having a baby, which are probably part of an evolutionary *protection* system, as you adjust to the responsibilities of parenting
- Believing that the thoughts mean something terrible about you, or what you will do, causes anxiety
- Trying to control your thoughts and taking other precautions keeps you in a cycle of anxiety
- Many factors including sleep deprivation, feelings of responsibility, high standards and past experiences can influence responding to unwanted intrusive thoughts (to try to get rid of them) in ways that can actually make them more persistent
- Understanding what the thoughts really are and practising not responding to the thoughts will help you to feel better

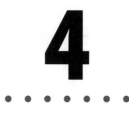

4

Specific Phobias Affecting Pregnancy and the Postnatal Period

---

In this chapter you will learn:

➤ What a phobia is and why we get them
➤ Particular features of the phobias that have special relevance for pregnancy, birth and early parenthood: phobia of vomiting (emetophobia) and phobia of blood, injuries and needles
➤ Practical strategies for dealing with these phobias to help you feel more in control and better able to manage situations when your phobia is triggered

---

NB: Two other phobias have particular importance in the perinatal period, which we cover elsewhere: tokophobia (fear of childbirth) is covered in Chapter 8 on pregnancy-related anxiety and social phobia (fear of being judged in social situations) is covered in Chapter 9 on adjusting to parenthood.

What Are Phobias?

A phobia is the experience of excessive and persistent anxiety or disgust triggered by a particular situation or set of related situations. Collectively, phobias are the most common form of anxiety disorder. Phobias can be about a range of topics, but commonly they are found around themes related to animals (or insects), blood and injury, situations (such as heights, crowded places, being in small places such as lifts, driving or flying), or others such as dental phobias, fears of choking or vomiting. Phobias of any type can of course coincide with the time of pregnancy and early parenthood, but two phobias have *particular* relevance to this period. These are emetophobia – a distressing fear of vomiting, and blood-injury-needle phobia, a fear of either directly experiencing or encountering triggers related to injury or medical procedures that can cause anxiety but also causes a very particular response of fainting.

If you have a phobia, you will know that it is much more than a dislike or aversion and causes distress and interference in your life. Encountering the thing you fear will always trigger distress and for some, a phobia can be so severe that even hearing related words or seeing a picture of what frightens them can cause anxiety or a fainting response. Often people go to extensive measures to avoid contact with what they fear and they become very good at organising life around this.

This may be manageable until normal life changes in some important way, such as becoming pregnant or a new parent. The majority of phobias, for example a fear of spiders, may not be heightened much in these new circumstances. However, others, such as fears of vomiting and fears of blood-injury have very direct relevance for pregnant and postnatal women. A well-known side effect of being pregnant is some experience of nausea or vomiting, estimated to occur in 50–90% of pregnancies. A small proportion of women (0.5–2%) suffer from hyperemesis, that is, being repeatedly sick during the pregnancy. In severe cases, women need hospital care to maintain hydration. This condition is unpleasant and difficult to cope with for anyone, but if you have a pre-existing phobia of vomiting, the very idea that this could happen, however unlikely, is very distressing. Indeed, some women feel that they are not able to contemplate pregnancy at all due to the strength of this fear and may very consciously delay or avoid pregnancy, even if having a child is very wanted. Any parent will confirm that looking after a small child involves contact with pretty much all their bodily fluids at some point. If you have emetophobia, you might be worried about whether this means an increased likelihood of being sick yourself due to concerns about catching bugs, or you may be worried about how your fears will impact your ability to look after your baby if they become ill and vomit.

For those with blood-injury phobia, becoming pregnant means that it is no longer possible to completely avoid triggers for your phobia. For your own safety and that of your baby, blood tests are necessary at various points in the pregnancy so that you can be provided with the best obstetric care. Some conditions, such as a difference in blood group between you and your baby (rhesus negative and rhesus positive), require an injection at birth for your safety to prevent disease. These interventions are very effective, but if you are a person with a longstanding blood-injury phobia, the idea of going through these procedures may feel very challenging.

The good news is that there are a range of techniques that you can use to combat these phobias and there is excellent evidence that these can really help.

What Causes Phobias?

About 7% of people suffer from a phobia during their lifetime, with fears of heights and animals being the most common. Phobias are more common in women, with the exception of blood-injury phobia which affects women and men equally. Emetophobia (a fear of vomiting) is thought to be significantly more common in women.

Generally, phobias begin in childhood or adolescence and can last through life if left untreated. Childhood is a time of making sense of all sorts of threat, and fears are very commonplace, with the type of fear mirroring our stage of development. Fears of separation are the first we experience, then animals, then more complex fears concerning illness and social fears. We tend to remember the first time we do things, so if you had a bad first experience, or a particularly traumatic encounter during this time, this sets up strong expectations about what this thing is like in general. This could be an aggressive dog barking at you as an infant, or a painful trip to the dentist. However, not all people with phobias have such a key learning experience that they remember.

Sometimes early experiences may be associated with other, more complex emotions than fear. Research into emetophobia has found that it is common to have strong aversive memories of early experiences of being sick, often accompanied by negative feelings, for example of not being cared for or looked after at the time. Often connections with a past experience may not be immediately obvious. There is something very primal about most phobias, in that people are aware that they are irrational and excessive, but when they are triggered, the physical response and drive to escape and avoid is very strong. It can be hard to express exactly what the fear is and so 'rationalise' it.

Fears are very common in childhood and usually they are transient and diminish over time. However, sometimes they persist and intensify. They can be enhanced by direct or indirect messages from parents, siblings or wider society, reinforcing the idea that a particular thing is scary and to be avoided. Being told or shown that some things are scary has a powerful impact when we are young. We are good at using social information to help us learn so we can benefit from the collective knowledge of the group, and so we use information from others to work out whether things are threatening or safe. We call this process 'social referencing'. For example, if your parent is making anxious faces at the idea of a spider being in the room, you may process this as important information about spiders.

Furthermore, how the people around you responded to your fear once it started can also embed anxiety. Parents who encourage avoidance and give a child the message that they would not be able to cope with danger or feelings of anxiety can inadvertently add to fears. Often parents themselves had these experiences and so have the same fears. The good news is that these cycles can be broken in two key ways: by working on your own fears and working on modelling confident responses with your own children, even if you don't feel completely confident (see Chapter 9 for more on adjusting to parenthood).

There is also likely a genetic element to phobias. Some people are more sensitive to feelings of anxiety, and are therefore susceptible to developing them if other circumstances are also present, such as those above. Genetic heritability varies depending on the type of phobia. Blood-injury phobia has the highest, followed by animal phobias and situational phobias (being in specific situations such as flying, driving, or being in enclosed spaces). If you have blood-injury phobia, you are probably able to think of a relative or two who shares this concern.

Blood-injury Phobia Is Different from Other Phobias: Fainting

All phobias and anxiety problems are associated with 'arousal' – a racing heart, faster breathing, alertness – as part of the survival mechanism to quickly escape danger ('flight'), or to be prepared to 'fight' (see Chapter 1 for more details). Blood-injury phobia is unique amongst phobias in that it is characterised by fainting, in which your heart rate and blood pressure drop after an initial rise (termed a vasovagal reaction). This response is also a part of our threat system, the last 'f' – fight, flight, freeze or *faint*. The theory is that this is a 'play dead' response that could be useful in situations of threat to our lives. The problem is that this evolutionarily advantageous response has outlived its usefulness in modern times, when it is activated by things like having an injection or seeing blood. With any type of anxiety problem, it is not due to any sort of defect or failing in the person. Yet often people with blood-injury phobias are made to feel as though they are somehow 'weak' or unable to cope due to their reactions. This is completely unfair. It's just luck of the draw to have this genetic makeup. Often people don't have the information that this is a specific phobia. It can feel like it's just 'part of who they are' and make them buy into the idea that it's a 'defect'. Unfortunately, this just leaves them suffering and stops them getting help for what is a very treatable problem.

KEY IDEA

Some people are more genetically prone to blood-injury phobia and associated fainting – it is not a character fault.

Pregnancy-specific Issues

Lissa: Blood and Injury Phobia

Lissa was 10 weeks pregnant and had been looking forward to getting to the second trimester. So far everything had been going well with the pregnancy. However, she was filled with fear about the blood test she knew she would have to take.

Since childhood, Lissa had been a 'fainter' at the sight of blood. This first became apparent when she had her Rubella and then BCG injections at school, both of which had caused her to faint in the nurse's office. They were horrible experiences – when the needle was brought out, before she knew much about it, she had felt like she was behind a black curtain and fell to the floor, waking up what felt like minutes later in a cold sweat, feeling weak and shaky as she recovered. The feeling was quickly overtaken by embarrassment, as she realised what had happened and was desperate to leave the room.

After this, friends and family would tease her about her 'squeamishness', and Lissa felt that it was a real weakness. She was of course keen to avoid any repeat of the situation. Generally, this was quite successful – Lissa managed to not have any injections at all, and avoided going to the doctor as much as possible. However, there were other times when she was unexpectedly exposed to gory material and had a similar reaction, for example when a friend who didn't know about her phobia showed her some pictures of an operation she had had. All this was manageable until Lissa became pregnant and she knew she could no longer avoid her fears.

OVER TO YOU
Do You Have a Blood-injury Phobia and How Does It Affect You?

Do you have an intense reaction of fear, disgust or fainting when you come into contact with (or anticipate):

Blood (or blood like substances, e.g. red paint or ketchup)
Physical injuries
Needles
Injections
Medical procedures and examinations
Pictures or discussions that remind you of the nature of human bodies or mortality

Do you tend to go out of your way to avoid situations that involve blood, injuries or injections? What situations do you tend to avoid?

Is your problem affecting your quality of life or relationships?

Moving Forward: How to Tackle Blood-injury Phobia with Applied Tension

As with most anxiety problems, the way to deal with this phobia is to approach what you have been avoiding. Unlike other anxiety problems, you need to do this while you apply a particular technique in order to override the fainting response. This technique is called *applied tension* (AT) and was developed by Professor Lars Goran-Ost in the early 1980s. The basic idea is that, by systematically squeezing your large muscles, you keep your blood pressure raised and thereby combat the physiological response of fainting. If you practise the technique, and then do it while exposing yourself to situations that make you feel dizzy, your body will learn to override the fainting reaction.

Step 1: Practise

Sit in a nice big chair like an armchair.

Tense the muscles of your arms, torso and legs and keep this going for 10–15 seconds, just long enough to feel warmth rising in your face. If this is hard, imagine yourself as a body builder striking a pose to make their muscles look massive. Then release the tension back to normal (but not to a relaxed state).

After 20–30 seconds, repeat and release. Do this five times. Practise five times per day for about a week before trying to combine this with exposure in step 2.

Step 2: Apply the Technique in the Situation that Makes You Feel Faint

Build up a hierarchy of triggers from mild to more challenging. Apply the technique as you gradually let yourself look at triggers or engage in situations that you would usually avoid (this is called 'exposure'). Start with the least fearful and try to tune into any early warning signs such as feeling a bit lightheaded. Engage in AT as soon as you feel any of these signs. Even if you feel faint, doing AT will help your reactions be less severe or long-lasting.

Lissa's list looked like this:

1. Thinking about blood
2. Look at a picture of a scab
3. Look at a picture of an operation
4. Watching a clip of a person breaking their leg
5. Watching a clip of a minor operation
6. Holding a syringe
7. Having an injection
8. Giving blood

A well-conducted scientific trial of AT with pregnant women who learned this technique in a group found that this was helpful in reducing fears, and the effects lasted into the postnatal period without any further treatment. AT has been found to be very effective, even when learned and practised in a single session, and it is thought to be very long-lasting [1]. You are likely to have lots of physical exams, blood tests and possibly other interventions in pregnancy. This technique can be practised now and used before each of these experiences to counteract the faint response. You will not faint in labour as your body will be contracting and effectively doing AT for itself!

Emetophobia: Why Do We Vomit?

Vomiting is a useful biological function to get rid of a potentially or actually harmful material from our bodies. It elicits feelings of disgust, which is a helpful emotion for survival, as it reinforces the message that anything that leaves your body shouldn't go back in. Animals that can't vomit, such as rats, are susceptible to poisoning.

The process of vomiting is an automatic response by our bodies, over which we can exercise some control – there is often time to run to the toilet or grab something to be sick in, but it's pretty hard to keep the vomit in once it has decided to come out. Not everyone finds vomiting frightening or disgusting, and there are individual differences between people in how they experience seeing others vomit, and vomiting themselves. You may know people who routinely deal with vomit in their everyday lives (e.g. working as a carer or in a school) or people who find vomiting funny. To overcome this problem, you don't have to be as carefree as them, but it is a good plan to move somewhat in that direction, in order to stop this problem from interfering with your pregnancy and being a parent.

Fear of Vomiting

Rhiannon

Rhiannon had been very worried about pregnancy. She had avoided it for years due to a longstanding fear of being sick. She knew it wasn't 'rational' and found it hard to explain to others, but somehow for her she felt that being sick was the worst thing that could happen. The idea of it filled her with dread and disgust and a sense that she couldn't cope.

She wanted to have children and so decided that she would take the chance and try for a baby with her partner Frank. Luckily the pregnancy had gone smoothly – although she had felt nauseous at times this had not developed into vomiting. She was excessively careful about what she ate and drank in pregnancy, sticking to her 'safe foods'. These were things which were not associated with food poisoning such as bread and potatoes. She had refused to eat anything she had not made herself during the pregnancy.

Postnatally things had gone well but her baby Barney was now eight months old and Rhiannon was quite limited in the range of foods she was feeding him, finding it hard to cook things she associated with vomiting illnesses like chicken. She was dreading settling him into nursery in a few months and the possible exposure to sickness bugs. She felt very guilty that her main fear was for herself being ill. She wasn't sure how she would cope if Barney was sick or worse still, if she picked something up. Rhiannon coped by having very high standards of hygiene and was constantly cancelling activities if she thought someone there might be ill. She closely monitored Barney and her husband for signs of illness.

What Keeps a Fear of Vomiting Going?

What You Believe About Vomiting: Awfulness and Likelihood

At the heart of emetophobia is the idea that being sick would be unbearably awful. Some people might even say they would prefer to die than vomit. If you believe this, it is understandable that you will spend a lot of your energy trying to avoid it. Some beliefs related to emetophobia include:

- If the baby starts vomiting, I will immediately vomit and I won't be able to cope, meaning I can't look after the baby
- If I have morning sickness and vomit, I will not be able to cope and will not be able to leave the house, I'll lose my job and I won't have any money

- If I have to go into a hospital for a pregnancy check or to give birth, I will pick up a vomiting bug and I will be ill for a long time
- If I start vomiting, I will not be able to stop and I will die (and my baby will be ill or die, or be left without a parent)
- If I start vomiting, I will get seriously ill and will be admitted to hospital; I will feel out of control and pick up more vomiting bugs, which will trap me in an endless cycle of vomiting
- If I start vomiting, I will shame myself in public and I will never get over it
- If I vomit in front of others, they will be angry or disgusted
- If I vomit, I will be vulnerable and I can't risk that
- If I can't cope with morning sickness or if I am frightened of going into hospital, then other people will judge me and think that I am weak

Sometimes your fears might be associated with a vivid image of what this would look like for you – how you would appear to others, and what reaction others would have to your vomiting.

Being sick isn't actually very common, but people with emetophobia over-estimate the risk, and so feel that all their efforts are successful and necessary. People with emetophobia become experts at avoiding situations which they feel might increase the likelihood of vomiting, such as being around people who could be ill due to bugs. Whilst no one particularly wants to be around people who are vomiting due to alcohol or motion sickness, this is often less threatening for someone with emetophobia as the cause is not contagious.

OVER TO YOU
What Is the Worst Thing About Vomiting for You?

If you can't think of anything other than 'it's disgusting', then this could be good news – you can build up your tolerance of vomit / vomiting in small steps. However, even if you can't identify any other 'worst thing', then read on as you will understand more about how this problem persists.

What You Do and What You Avoid

If you are anxious about vomiting, you may take a number of precautions to prevent the worst from happening. You may scan yourself or others for signs of sickness in order to catch the situation early or spend a lot of time trying to plan or mentally prepare for being sick or coping if someone else is sick (including your baby). You might ask for lots of reassurance that someone you are with isn't ill, or you may spend a lot of time checking food and ingredients to make sure it is safe. You might avoid situations which you feel raise the risk of vomiting or contact with vomit, e.g. public toilets, visiting people who are ill, eating food in particular situations (e.g. when it is cooked by someone else).

As with any fear, this combination of avoidance and hypervigilance (excessive attention) to signs in your body or the outside world that something could trigger vomiting, make the fear feel more real.

There is lots of detail in the chapter on intrusive thoughts about exactly how avoidance and other behaviours operate to keep anxiety going (see Chapter 3). A summary is provided here.

Response to the thought that you will be sick and this will be unbearable in some way	What you are trying to do	What is the unintended consequence
Monitor yourself and others for signs of being ill	Catch any early warning signs so you are prepared	Makes you feel like very normal sensations are a sign that you might be ill and keeps you focused on threat
Avoidance of particular situations or people	Reduce the chances of being ill	Stops you finding out that this would not happen anyway, even if you did not avoid the situation

Response to the thought that you will be sick and this will be unbearable in some way	What you are trying to do	What is the unintended consequence
Reassurance	Trying to be certain you won't be ill	Increases doubt and makes you less sure. Fuels the idea that you cannot cope
Focus on early bad experience	Remind yourself of how bad it is and how important it is to avoid	Makes you forget that you survived this experience and you have likely developed and matured your ability to cope in many ways since
Excessive washing	Trying to ensure you won't be ill	Stops you finding out that this would not happen anyway and gives you sore hands
Only eating particular foods or in particular situations	Trying to ensure you won't be ill	Stops you finding out this would not happen anyway even if you ate it
Plan how you would cope if self or others were sick	Feel like you can cope	Undermines your confidence you can cope and makes you feel like this is likely
Carry anti-emetic medication or other precautions, e.g. water, sick bag etc.	Feel like you can cope	Undermines your confidence you can cope and makes you feel like this is likely
Avoid thinking about vomit as it might make it more likely (magical thinking)	Try to prevent vomiting	Buys into the idea that you are at risk of vomiting
Anxiety, disgust	Keeps you alert to dealing with danger and feels like it's telling you something	Is kept going by all of the above

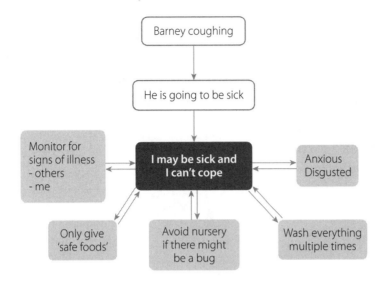

The average age for onset of emetophobia is about nine. It is not a coincidence that many people with this problem report negative early experiences of either them or another person vomiting in childhood. The experience is usually negative in terms of the emotion that was felt at the time. This could be fear or disgust due to the suddenness of the event, or how it was dealt with by adults, such as being made to feel ashamed or weak. It also might be associated with other aspects of the original circumstances, like being a long way from home, trapped or being associated with a time of stress such as moving school or home, bereavement or parental marital breakdown.

Here is Rhiannon's example.

> Rhiannon had a clear memory of being 8 years old and at home with her younger sister after school one day watching TV. She recalled suddenly feeling ill and being sick in the living room, vomiting some lurid pink biscuits she had recently eaten. Her mother burst into the room and shouted at her for making a mess, making her feel sad and ashamed.

For some people, part of avoiding being sick is in some way an attempt to avoid painful negative emotions that were linked with the experience at a young age. These connections might not be at the front of your mind on the everyday level, but if you had a bad experience like this, it may be playing a role in what makes the idea of being sick so scary.

OVER TO YOU
What Factors Are Keeping My Problem Going?

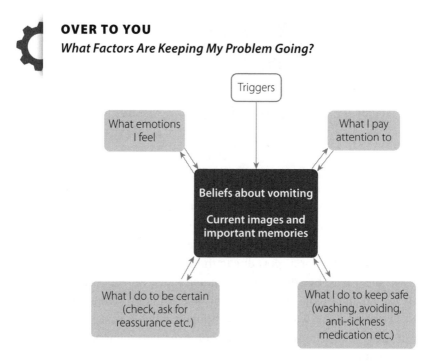

Reset Your Goals

All phobias cause interference in life. Even if you find clever ways of managing them, it takes effort and is at best inconvenient, especially if you are trying to also manage the demands of pregnancy or caring for a young baby. Usually, the cost to you will be much greater than this when you factor in what you can and can't do, your quality of life and your relationships.

It's worth thinking for a moment about the difficulties the problem has been causing you and what you would like to change.

Think about how you would like things to be different and what the first steps might be to getting there.

Moving Forward: Treating Emetophobia as an Anxiety Problem

Somewhere along the line you have absorbed the idea that:

1. Vomiting is likely, and that
2. If it happened, it would unbearably awful and you would not cope.

Let's call this idea 'Theory A'.

It makes sense therefore that you are doing everything you can to avoid it. The alternative is that neither of these ideas is true, but that you have developed an excessive fear that needs dealing with for you to be able to live your life in a less restricted and stressful way. Let's call this idea 'Theory B'.

We will compare these two theories and work out which one best fits with your experiences; first thinking about what fits with each idea, then considering what kinds of behaviours go along with each one. See p. 71 for further examples of Theory A, Theory B.

Rhiannon's completed table is shown below.

Theory A	Theory B
The problem is it is (highly) likely I will be nauseous and sick; this will be awful and I will not cope = A VOMITING PROBLEM	I have developed a fear of being sick – I overestimate how likely and how awful it will be and underestimate how able I would be to cope with it if it happened = A FEAR OF VOMITING PROBLEM

Theory A	Theory B
Why do I believe this? It feels very likely – I often feel a bit nauseous	Even if it 'feels' likely, that doesn't mean it is actually going to happen I am very focused on how I feel, and feel more sick as a result of being so tuned into tiny changes in my body I think I have been caught in the 'using feelings as evidence' trap – taking feeling bad as evidence that something bad is going to happen
Just don't think I can deal with it	In reality, I have coped well when others are sick I can cope with lots of other things, like others being injured, without difficulty I have a demanding job which people say I'm good at I don't have to be 'brilliant' or 'the best' at coping, I just have to be able to deal with it at the time – nobody really likes dealing with vomit or vomiting, everyone just puts up with it
When I was sick, aged 8, my mum was angry	Looking back, I realise she probably had emetophobia too, and she was upset and anxious. As I didn't realise this at the time, this might partly explain why I have developed a fear, as I was so upset and distressed by vomiting and her anger
What do I need to do if this is true? Do everything possible not to be sick Check people for signs of illness and avoid them Avoid eating chicken, fish etc. Washing	Drop all the extra precautions I have been doing Face my fears, not avoid them, and even approaching scenarios where someone might be sick Remember that I'm not more likely to be sick or less able to cope with it than anyone else. No one likes it but it's a necessary bodily function

Theory A	Theory B
What happens if I carry on doing these things? Not much fun Restricted life for me and Barney Continued stress as he goes to nursery and then to school	It should get easier over time and I should feel less afraid

OVER TO YOU

Your Theory A versus Theory B

Consider the questions below to help you compare the evidence that actually supports each idea, and the strategies that go along with each alternative.

Theory A	Theory B
The problem is it is (highly) likely I will be nauseous and sick; this will be awful and I will not cope = A VOMITING PROBLEM	**I have developed a fear of being sick – I overestimate how likely and how awful it will be and underestimate how able I would be to cope with it if it happened = A FEAR OF VOMITING PROBLEM**
Why do I believe this? **What do I need to do if this is true?**	
What happens if I carry on doing these things?	

Experimenting with Doing Things Differently: Putting Theory to the Test

Rhiannon decided to test out her idea that she or her baby would get ill if they ate chicken. She couldn't face cooking chicken, but still tried to really challenge herself:

Complete before the experiment		Complete after the experiment		
What will I do?	**What am I testing out?**	**Did my predictions come true?**	**What did I find out?**	**Does this fit best with Theory A or Theory B?**
Give Barney some pre-prepared chicken baby food	He will get ill (50% likely) I will get ill too (50% likely) I will be unwell for several days (100% likely) I will not cope – meaning I will not be able to look after Barney (100%)	After 3–4 hours – no After 12 hours – no After 34 hours – no After 48 hours – no 0% getting ill	He did not get ill, even though he ate chicken	Theory B – I have been treating chicken as if it was poison Barney needs to eat protein and he liked it

Rhiannon built on this task by giving him different chicken dishes such as prepared roasted chicken, breaded chicken sticks, chicken and rice – she worked her way up to preparing chicken herself. This was difficult as she was very preoccupied with the raw chicken and whether it had touched anything. She did it, but it took a long time and it was stressful. She asked her brother to come and help her, and to point out to her if she was doing anything 'extra' in the preparation or clearing up that was motivated by avoiding vomit-related illness rather than what most people would do when cooking chicken. This went well and boosted her confidence that she could do it again on her own.

OVER TO YOU
Testing Things Out

Hopefully by mapping out your vicious flower and Theory A versus Theory B table, you will have noticed that all the additional precautions you have been taking to manage your fears are actually playing a role in keeping them going.

Dropping these behaviours and doing the things you have been avoiding is the way to start to overcome them. Some examples of common experiments are going without anti-emetic medication, having a chicken sandwich, taking a bus, watching a video of a person vomiting.

Complete before the experiment		Complete after the experiment		
What will I do?	What am I testing out?	Did my predictions come true?	What did I find out?	Does this fit best with Theory A or Theory B?

Tackling Frightening Images Associated with Vomiting

Do you have a recurrent image or memory that comes to mind when you feel fearful of vomiting? We know that images like this are common when people feel anxious and often connect either in content or in meaning to a difficult past experience associated with vomiting. Sometimes they might be triggered by situations that overlap in some way with your past experience and consequently remind you of that past threat.

Images are important to consider as, just like anxious thoughts, they may be part of what is keeping your anxiety about vomiting going. They may amplify your sense of threat around vomit or they might pull you into taking unhelpful precautions. The good news is that, just like anxious thoughts, they can be tackled.

Rhiannon had a recurrent image of being curled up, helpless on the floor in a vast flood of vomit. She linked this to the clear memory she had of being 8 years old and vomiting suddenly on the living room floor. During that incident she also felt helpless, ashamed and afraid and shocked at how much vomit there was. She remembers cowering as her mum shouted at her.

OVER TO YOU

First focus on the emotion you feel when you imagine vomiting. What images do you experience? Can you close your eyes and imagine it for a moment? What do you see? What is happening? How are you feeling in the image?

Are there aspects of this image which appear to link to difficult past experiences of vomiting? Perhaps the way you look, feel or behave in the image, the way vomit appears to you or the ways others are reacting?

Have you noticed particular triggers to the image? Do they seem to match some aspect of your past experience in some way, e.g. when you see or smell particular things, or when you are in particular places?

The worst thing for Rhiannon about the image was the amount of vomit she could see and the sense of helplessness and shame she was feeling. The image made her think vomiting would always be horrific, that she would be helpless to do anything, and that people wouldn't help – only criticise her. She also feared that vomiting would go on forever and that she would be surrounded by a huge lake.

What is the worst thing about the image for you? What does it say about vomit? What does it say about you as a person and your ability to cope? What does it say about other people and how they might intervene?

Rhiannon looked at the evidence for the meaning attached to her image, i.e. the belief 'Vomiting will always be horrific and go on forever, I will be helpless and people will criticise me', which she believed to be 90% true when she was feeling her most anxious. Some of her evidence is shown below:

Evidence for the idea	Other ways of looking at this
The vomit in the living room was huge and felt like it went on forever	It probably looked huge to me because I was little. I know from spilling Barney's milk that even a tiny bit looks big on the floor. Even though it felt like it went on forever, it did stop.
I've heard lots of people say how 'gross' it is when they see someone being sick	Vomit might be disgusting but it is a normal, protective bodily function. It doesn't make me disgusting as a person.
The living room incident was horrific	It was a horrible experience but it was my first time being very sick and mum was unfair on me. I haven't been sick like that since, so I don't have much experience to draw on. Other people seem to manage being sick okay.
Mum shouted at me	She was angry about her new carpet and tired after work. When I've asked her about it since she says she is sorry for shouting at me as she knew I couldn't help it. She is also afraid of vomiting. I know Heston at least isn't the kind of person to criticise me and he has often helped his friends when they weren't well on a night out.

What is your evidence for the meaning attached to your image? Like Rhiannon, can you think of any other ways of looking at it?

Evidence for the idea	Other ways of looking at this

Rhiannon considered how she could summarise the other ways of looking at her evidence:

> Vomit is disgusting, but that doesn't make me a disgusting person. If it did, everyone would be disgusting! A small amount can look like a lot. Vomiting is unpleasant but it does stop. It is possible there are ways of managing and I know Heston would help me.

How could you summarise the other ways of looking at your evidence?

Rhiannon then thought about how she could transform her anxiety-provoking image to fit with her new ways of looking at things. She closed her eyes and brought to mind her image. First, she imagined her partner and her good friend coming into the image. She imagined them walking over to her and asking if she was okay in a warm tone of voice. Her partner laid a hand on her back. She also saw her mum come in saying 'I'm so sorry, are you okay?'. She imagined herself uncurling and standing up tall, the pool of vomit shrinking down as she did so. She saw herself wiping her mouth and walking over to a comfortable chair where she sits down and drinks some water.

Just as Rhiannon did, is there a way to transform your image to fit your new ways of looking at things? What would need to change? Would you bring someone into the image with you? Would you change the size and shape of anything or how you behaved? Try to experiment with the image until you notice a shift in how threatening it feels.

OVER TO YOU
Keeping It Going

It is really important to make a plan to keep challenging your phobia of vomit. Emetophobia is very often a longstanding problem and you need to keep working on it to make Theory B your 'new normal'. Keeping a note of the experiments you have done and what you have learnt, together with your next steps, can help. Don't worry if a challenging situation occurs and you find it difficult, such as someone suddenly being taken ill near you. Most of us find some aspects of these situations difficult. Try to focus on what you did well and be kind to yourself about the additional challenge someone with emetophobia has to deal with in these circumstances. Plan to do more experiments to claim back your everyday life. This is more important than these rare events.

We know that applied tension works very well and if you keep doing it for a consistent period alongside exposure, it seems that the fainting response can be largely overcome. People with this phobia might not ever enjoy the idea of blood and gore, but once they have practised applied tension, people often find that further experiences of fainting are rare. It will always be something you can practise if you need to ahead of anything you find triggering, such as injections etc.

To Sum Up

- A phobia is the repeated experience of intense anxiety or fainting in response to a *specific* situation or set of triggers
- Applied tension is a simple technique that works very well to counteract the fainting response in blood-injury-injection phobia
- Fear of vomiting is a serious anxiety problem in which the likelihood and awfulness of vomiting is overestimated, and coping is radically underrated
- You can beat this fear by challenging these beliefs actively, dropping safety behaviours like excessive washing, limiting diet and approaching situations you fear
- Early experiences often play a role in keeping the fear going and the meaning and emotion in those memories can be updated

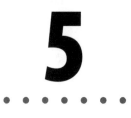

Panic Attacks and Health Worries

In this chapter you will learn:

➤ What a panic attack is and why they happen

➤ Why the situation of pregnancy and the postnatal period might make them more likely

➤ How our attention, beliefs about what is happening, and how we act on those beliefs play a key role in panic attacks and worries about health

➤ Techniques to gain a new understanding of physical sensations in panic and health worries

➤ How to apply these tools to feel better about your health

In this chapter we are focused on physical sensations in your body, what they mean to you, and how what you believe about those physical feelings has led to anxiety about your health and panic.

Please continue to follow the advice of your midwife, doctor and other qualified health professionals who know the specifics of your health and pregnancy. It is fine to ask them questions for reassurance. If you are asking repeatedly you may want to discuss with them the other techniques described in this chapter.

Understanding Strong Physical Sensations of Panic

OVER TO YOU

Is Panic a Problem for You?

Do you:

- Have sudden, very intense anxiety attacks, that come out of the blue?
- Worry about physical sensations in your body such as changes in your heart rate, changes in your breathing, dizziness or lightheadedness, changes in temperature, nausea (or any other sensation that frightens you)?
- Feel constantly concerned about having panic attacks?
- Avoid situations or circumstances that you fear may lead to a panic attack?
- Has this problem started to get in the way of your normal day-to-day life?

What Do these Physical Sensations Mean?

Physical feelings in our bodies change all the time for an untold number of reasons. Can you think of a time when you had to give a speech or a presentation to a large number of people? Or a time when you have waited for an exam result, or before you took your driving test? Or do you remember when you found out that you were pregnant or first felt your baby move? On any of these occasions, did you feel your heart race, feel your skin prickle, feel very hot, get a shiver down your spine, feel a little breathless, or feel a lurch in your stomach? Whether finding out you were pregnant was an experience ranging from overwhelmingly positive, through to underwhelming ordinary, or even a stressful experience, it is almost certain that you had a physical response to some degree. The physical experiences of a racing heart, breathlessness, or other strong sensations in your body may have been associated with excitement, trepidation or shock, and would have dissipated after a short while as you took the news in. There was a clear context for understanding what was going on, a reason for feeling those things. The point is, different events and contexts provoke a state of 'arousal' in our bodies (not meaning sexual arousal, but an overall state of alertness that prepares our bodies and minds to react quickly and to optimise our performance – see Chapter 1). This state of arousal can be part of excitement or anticipation, or apprehension and fear, even when the sensations are quite similar. However, if the link between the sensation and the context is not clear, you may think something terrible is happening, which is obviously a very scary thought. This may also affect what you then do, what you notice and what you then believe is happening – see the table on page 119.

KEY IDEA

Sensations such as a racing heart, breathlessness or dizziness are normal. If you interpret these sensations as a sign of something bad happening, you may experience panic.

Why Do I Notice These Sensations?

The vast majority of physical sensations we experience are harmless bodily functions or fluctuations, e.g. our guts being more or less active, our eyes feeling tired, aches and pains. Sometimes these changes are very noticeable and capture your attention – if you then interpret that feeling as a sign of something bad happening in your body, it's not surprising that you feel extremely anxious and panicky. If you have had a panic attack or other experience, you may be more tuned into the sensations, so that they come into your awareness even at very low levels. Therefore, the interpretations are activated very easily, causing more anxiety and also fuelling more sensations.

Same feelings, different interpretations

Context	Physical feeling	Interpretation / what you believe about that feeling or sensation	What emotion you experience	What you do	What do you find out?
Walking up the stairs on a hot day, when you are tired and out of sorts	Trembling Heart racing Sweating Shallow breathing	I'm having a stroke I'm having a heart attack I'm about to radically overheat and have a fit I'm suffocating	Panic, anxiety	Stop Seek reassurance Avoid stairs Avoid all exercise	That even if I try and avoid all physical sensations, I still experience some, and I worry all the time about having a panic attack and believe that something bad is going to happen
Giving a speech at your sister's wedding	Trembling Heart racing Sweating Shallow breathing	I'm so nervous about getting this right as it's such a special day	Anxiety	Give the speech	That the feelings of anxiety passed and I could do it
Having an enjoyable day out at a funfair, going on the rollercoaster	Trembling Heart racing Sweating Shallow breathing	This is fun	Excitement	Keep going on rollercoaster	I had a thrilling time

This panic cycle was identified by David Clark (1985) [1] and is the basis of extremely effective CBT:

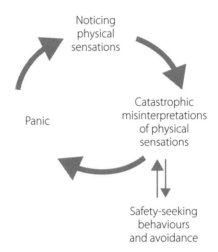

Noticing the sensations in your body is not the problem. Some people are more aware of their heart rate and other feelings in their body than others – it's just something that varies between individuals, e.g. some athletes are very tuned into their bodies and might be able to notice very slight changes, but this would signal interest rather than fear.

KEY IDEA

Once you regard sensations in your body as a sign of something bad happening, you will notice them more – your attention is quickly directed to the sensations.

We all pay attention to things that feel more important to us – see the bird scurvy metaphor on page 58. What this means for you is that you may be more aware of e.g. your heart rate, but you may or may not be accurate at *interpreting* what you feel. Remember anxiety can shift our thinking patterns. If there is something ambiguous or uncertain going on in your body (was that a missed beat? Is my breathing becoming shallower?) then you may be more likely to interpret that as a sign of something very serious happening right now, bringing on the horrible feeling of impending disaster, leading to escalating anxiety and a panic attack. With health anxiety, you are likely to think that the health disaster is not imminent (i.e. happening right now, today e.g. I am having a stroke) but at some point in the future e.g. this could be a sign of cancer. The cycle is otherwise very similar in that the interpretations keep anxiety going.

Panic Attacks in the Context of Pregnancy and the Postnatal Period

The journey to motherhood causes huge changes in the body, and you will have noticed many sensations in your body that are new and different. Some of these sensations may feel very welcome, such as feeling your baby move, and can bring great happiness and excitement. Other sensations may concern you and provoke concerns about whether you or your baby is healthy. Having some worries or feeling very anxious for short periods of time is almost inevitable in pregnancy, as there are so many different physical changes, both expected and unexpected. You will have been given a lot of very general information and advice about pregnancy and probably been asked in a general way to monitor your physical symptoms, often without clear guidelines to follow. Most pregnancies do progress without problems, and routine monitoring by midwives or obstetricians can help to pick up and address potential problems. This chapter will help you if you have been very concerned about physical sensations in your body, believing them to mean that you (or your baby) are seriously unwell, and provoking extreme anxiety and panic.

If you are struggling with repeated panic attacks, when you notice an unusual sensation in your body, it will be difficult to remember what you know and understand when you are not anxious – that most sensations are normal and transient, and that it is likely that this feeling will pass. Panic attacks occur when you think that the physical feeling is a sign of danger to your health, and / or the health of your baby. Once you start thinking in this catastrophic way, you naturally start to feel more and more anxious, generating more and more physical sensations in your body, that further fuel frightening ideas about what is going on. Not surprisingly, you will try to do anything to get rid of the feelings of anxiety and to make yourself feel safer – this may include asking for reassurance from those around you or seeking emergency medical care. We call these strategies 'safety-seeking' behaviours.

Unfortunately, although most of these actions might have given you temporary reassurance or peace of mind, they do not help the panic problem to go away. You can feel like you've escaped, rather than solved the problem and live in fear of it happening again.

Panic Attacks in Pregnancy

Amana

Amana was 28 weeks pregnant and had been enjoying swimming and yoga, and had a few weeks left of work before going on maternity leave. She enjoyed socialising and being outside.

Her midwives were running a campaign on pre-eclampsia and she had been given a lot of information on physical health during pregnancy. She realised that she had some of the minor risk factors associated with pre-eclampsia, as she was over 40, and was told she was slightly overweight, although the charts used were not based on people from her ethnic group so she was uncertain whether this was valid information or not.

Amana had a straightforward pregnancy and her midwives were not concerned about pre-eclampsia or any other physical health condition for her. One day, whilst standing cooking in her kitchen, Amana suddenly noticed feeling breathless and very hot – she felt extremely anxious, and believed that she was developing pre-eclampsia and that she and her baby were about to die. She called an ambulance and was taken to hospital, where the medical team concluded that she was healthy, as was the baby. She was discharged that day and returned home feeling shocked and confused.

She bought her own blood pressure monitor but was too frightened to use it. She avoided cooking and other household tasks, and stayed at home as much as possible, trying to move slowly and never exert herself. If she was feeling anxious then she took deep breaths and tried to monitor her pulse. She asked her partner for reassurance that she was ok and that she was not harming their baby.

Panic Attacks Postnatally

Nuwa

Nuwa had a ten-week-old baby who was born at a slightly low weight, and both she and the baby had to stay in hospital for a week after the birth. When they were discharged, Nuwa felt quite disoriented at home, and often felt unreal or lightheaded.

One day, when she was looking at herself and the baby in the mirror, she felt very strange, as if she wasn't really there, and had an intense surge of panic. She believed that she was 'losing her mind' or 'going mad'. She put her baby down on the floor and rang her partner begging them to come home as soon as possible. Since then, she has avoided being on her own with the baby, and avoided looking in mirrors for fear of re-experiencing the same sensation. She often pinches herself to check that she still feels like she is real. She has spent a lot of time online looking up symptoms of schizophrenia, and constantly monitors herself for any change in how she is feeling.

A Note on Post-partum Psychosis

This is a rare form of severe mental illness that affects about 1/1000 mothers, usually starting in the first few days after birth. It has many features which are different from panic and anxiety and requires a different type of treatment. Some mothers experience some or all of the symptoms of hallucinations (hearing, seeing, smelling or feeling things that are not there), delusions, loss of inhibition, behaving out of character, feeling suspicious, confused and fearful, accompanied by changes in mood. These mood changes could be feeling really 'high', thinking and talking quickly, or feeling depressed, or a mixture of both. Symptoms can sometimes be hard to spot but are usually noticeably 'out of character' for the person. Immediate treatment by a specialist perinatal mental health team is available to help you recover as quickly as possible. If you are concerned that you or a loved one may be suffering from post-partum psychosis, please speak to your general health practitioner or maternity service as soon as possible. Out of their working hours you can get help and support either via 999 or at your local Accident and Emergency department. Post-partum psychosis is treatable and getting treatment early means you will make a full recovery more quickly.

Panic Attacks Related to Other Forms of Anxiety

Panic attacks can accompany other difficulties. If your panic attacks occur only in specific situations, you may find it helpful to read this chapter and other specific chapters in the book – see the table below for more information:

If you only feel very panicky or have panic attacks when you think of a past traumatic event.	See Chapter 7 on trauma.
If you only feel very panicky or have panic attacks at the thought of blood tests, injections.	See Chapter 4 on blood injury phobia.
If you only feel very panicky or have panic attacks when you have unwanted intrusive thoughts of harm or other unwanted thoughts, images or urges.	See Chapter 3 on unwanted intrusive thoughts of harm.
If you only feel very panicky or have panic attacks when thinking about birth.	See Chapter 8 on tokophobia.

What if you worry about or feel anxiety or panic when thinking about sensations in your body, but rather than worrying that it means you will die or come to serious harm right now, you worry that you are seriously ill with a disease that will cause your death or other life-changing outcome at some point in the future? You might have panic attacks or feel very panicky when you notice sensations in your body that you believe are a sign of future illness (e.g. a serious disease such as cancer, MS, motor neurone disease). When worries about illness are focused on the future, rather than something bad happening immediately, this can be understood as 'health anxiety' – which is sometimes referred to as hypochondriasis. You have probably heard the term 'hypochrondriac', which can be used to dismiss concerns or used as a perjorative label. Health anxiety or illness anxiety are usually more helpful ways to refer to this difficulty.

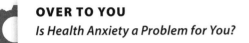

OVER TO YOU
Is Health Anxiety a Problem for You?

Do you:

- Constantly worry about your health
- Frequently check yourself for signs of something wrong (e.g. lumps)
- Very frequently ask people or check the Internet for reassurance that you are not seriously unwell
- Make frequent trips to the doctor to ask for tests – or avoid medical appointments all together
- Find that the problem persists or worsens despite reassurance from others, medical professionals or online sources, and impairs day-to-day life.

In terms of what people do to manage their doubts and fears, health anxiety can be very similar to OCD, which is described in Chapter 3. Continue reading this chapter, as how we understand panic is highly relevant to health anxiety, but you may also find the ideas in Chapter 3 on tackling unwanted intrusive thoughts useful too, particularly how asking for reassurance, repeated checking and avoiding activities can all be behaviours which keep these types of anxiety problems going. You may have experienced health anxiety in the past but at present your worry is more about the health of the baby or pregnancy-specific worries, in which case Chapter 8 on pregnancy-specific anxiety may also be of use.

What Keeps Panic Going? Background Factors

We know that people who suffer from panic attacks may be more sensitive to the physical manifestations of anxiety and find them more unpleasant than others. This is just part of the 'factory settings' we are all born with and may not be an issue unless it combines with other circumstances. Let's come back to the issue that panic attacks are a problem for you now, when you are pregnant or after you have had a baby (the perinatal period). It is understandable because this situation involves lots of physical change and challenges which may trigger symptoms for some. This seems to be more the case for first-time mothers, perhaps as the sensations are very new. Some women report an improvement in their symptoms of panic attacks if they had them before pregnancy, but for some it worsens or stays the same. There is a lot of variation and each individual pregnancy can be different, so it is hard to generalise about the effect of pregnancy on panic. The physical effect of changes in hormones means that the immediate postnatal period or stopping breastfeeding can be a time of increased vulnerability to panic, possibly by increasing relevant physical sensations such as body temperature, for example.

As well as physical changes in the perinatal period, the additional dimension of being responsible for a baby may also play a role in the awfulness of panic, and therefore how anxious it is making you feel: you might be doing anything to avoid having a panic attack, as you might be worried about harm coming to the baby from the panic itself, as well as what the impact of this anxiety could be on the baby (see Chapter 1 for more information on that).

You may have been given a lot of 'better safe than sorry' messages from health professionals about your own vulnerability and the baby's vulnerability – whilst these messages will have been well-intended, this may have reinforced the idea that there is something to worry about, and may have kept the focus of your attention on problems and worries, rather than on what is going well with your pregnancy, and what you don't need to worry about. Often, pregnant women are dealing with a number of very real stressors and juggling lots of things, like work, relationships, other caring responsibilities, finance and housing issues. This kind of stress can have an impact and almost certainly plays a role in anxiety issues. Looking after yourself as best you can and keeping the basics going (adequate sleep, feeding yourself) are really important.

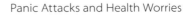

What Keeps Panic Going? Factors in the Present

In the rest of this chapter, you will find out how to stop panic being a problem for you. What you need to be on the lookout for is what you are doing to try to feel better, but how this might actually be making the problem worse. In CBT, we identify both cognitive (thinking) and behavioural (what you do) processes that keep the frightening idea or belief going that there is something wrong with your body and you are in danger of being seriously ill or dying.

Things You Do to Try and Stay Safe (Safety-seeking Behaviours and Avoidance)

As introduced in Chapter 1, when you believe that something bad is going to happen, it makes sense to avoid situations that trigger those thoughts and feelings, and to do things that you believe minimise the likelihood of the bad thing happening. However, unfortunately, avoiding this *perceived* risk stops you from finding out what actually happens. This is a really important idea and explains why physical sensations remain scary even when the bad thing doesn't happen. It's a bit like wearing garlic to keep away vampires. It definitely works because they haven't bitten yet, right?

So when you start to feel panicky, if you leave the situation, or do something to reduce the physical sensations, you lose the opportunity to learn that the sensations will pass whether or not you do anything, and that the awful outcome that you fear doesn't actually happen. However, you are left with the belief that the thing you did was crucial in saving you.

 KEY IDEA

Safety-seeking behaviours stop you finding out that the sensations aren't dangerous in the way you fear.

The following table contains some examples of how actions or decisions you might have taken to try to solve the perceived problem of imminent danger to your health actually have the opposite effect of keeping your beliefs, and therefore the panic problem, going:

What processes keep the problem going?	Examples	How the solution becomes the problem
Avoidance	Avoiding exercise	You may feel physically deconditioned or unfit, so taking any exercise can produce more physical sensations or discomfort
	Avoiding health appointments or information about health / pregnancy / post-childbirth	You miss out on the opportunity to get real, accurate information about your health
	Avoiding being alone	You lose confidence in your own judgement and abilities The more you avoid, the more you will want to avoid
Checking	Frequently taking pulse or blood pressure Checking online for information about health	Repeated checking or searching for information increases the feeling of doubt, uncertainty and anxiety
'Hypervigilance' to physical sensations	'Tuning in' to any small change in your body	The more attention you pay to e.g. a bodily sensation, the more you will notice it, and the less you will notice occasions when the sensation is absent
Selective attention ('cherry picking')	To news stories about illness or death in pregnant women / new mothers To information from health professionals that focuses on risk and worst-case scenarios	The harder you are 'looking for trouble', the more you will find information that appears to confirm your frightening ideas about your health
Reassurance seeking	Asking your partner or other relatives or friends questions about health or about what you should or shouldn't do	Repeated requests for reassurance increase the feeling of doubt, uncertainty and anxiety, and reduce your confidence in your own judgement

What processes keep the problem going?	Examples	How the solution becomes the problem
Other 'counter productive' strategies	E.g. taking deep breaths to try to 'control' breathing, or breathing into a paper bag	Deliberately trying to control your body brings your attention back to the sensations, and can often make them worse Your body will regulate itself if you leave it alone

You might get some temporary relief, but over time, it is likely that all this has taken up more time, and you have become more restricted in what you do.

You may have read about or been told to do breathing exercises to alleviate anxiety. For many years, people were advised to breathe into a paper bag if they felt panicky. Breathing exercises as part of relaxation can be helpful and bring about a wonderful state of calmness and well-being, and that might be something you have enjoyed. However, we are not recommending using breathing exercises or relaxation for overcoming panic, as trying to control physical sensations often makes them worse, and doing anything to change the physical sensations implies they are dangerous and must be managed or controlled to stop something bad happening to you. This is not the case.

Remember the panic cycle from earlier? Our thoughts or beliefs about the physical sensations in the moment move the experience of physical sensations into a panic attack. Think about times in your life when you have suddenly had to run – to catch a bus, or if something you were holding blew away in the wind. You might have felt breathless and your heart would have been racing, but did you need to lie and do a relaxation exercise to re-regulate your breathing? Or grab a paper bag and start counting your breaths? When we watch the Olympics, do the athletes recover after a race by deliberately controlling their breathing? No – they stand there and let their bodies work it out. Whilst you might not think your body looks similar to an Olympic athlete at the moment, the fundamental physiology of your body is exactly the same. In fact, many women have competed in the Olympics whilst pregnant – Martina Valcepina won a medal in speed skating whilst pregnant with twins.

If we consider Amana and Nuwa, we can see how what they do when they feel anxious reinforces their beliefs that something bad is happening:

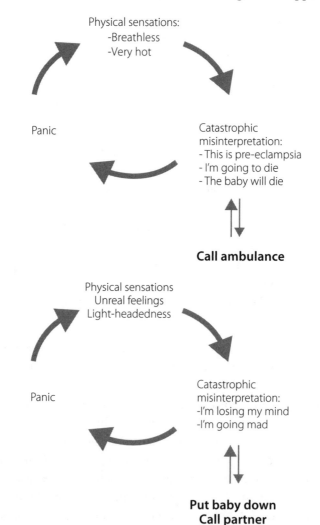

Moving Forward: Spotting Anxious Thinking in Panic

KEY IDEA

You don't feel the intense anxiety of a panic attack unless you are thinking that something terrible is happening or is going to happen.

Let's see how this works for Amana and Nuwa:

Amana

Questions to ask myself	
Last time I felt panicky or had a panic attack, what feelings in my body frightened me?	Breathlessness Feeling very hot
What was going through my mind? What's so bad about having that sensation? What's the worst thing that could happen? What images came into my mind?	This isn't right This is a sign of pre-eclampsia I will fall unconscious and die Image of myself in hospital, unresponsive, with medical team around me, my partner with a look of despair on their face
What do I do when I'm thinking this?	Stay still or move very slowly Try and take deep breaths Check my pulse and see if it is any quicker Check myself for other signs of high blood pressure Ask my partner for reassurance

Nuwa

Last time I felt panicky or had a panic attack, what feelings in my body frightened me?	Feeling dizzy and unreal
What was going through my mind?	I'm losing my mind, I'm going mad
What's so bad about having that sensation?	It will build up and up
What's the worst thing that could happen?	I'll lose control of myself
What images came into my mind?	Image of screaming and pulling at my hair, baby terrified and crying
What do I do when I'm thinking this?	Put the baby down Try to feel more real Pinch myself / dig my nails into my hands Look up symptoms of serious mental illness

OVER TO YOU

Understanding Your Panic Cycle

Take yourself back to a time in the last day or two when you have felt very anxious and panicky:

Questions to ask myself	
Last time I felt panicky or had a panic attack, what feelings in my body frightened me?	
What was going through my mind? **What's so bad about having that sensation?** **What's the worst thing that could happen?** **What images came into my mind?**	
What do I do when I'm thinking this	

Moving Forward: Understanding Your Problem as Anxiety

What you have read so far should help you to see that panic has persisted as a problem for you because you have believed that normal bodily sensations are more dangerous than they actually are, and that these interpretations or beliefs motivate and drive reactions which maintain the idea that something bad is happening, or even make it worse. You might 'know' that you are physically healthy (or no less healthy or at risk than anyone else) but you might 'feel' that it's too risky to go back to what you did before panic was a problem for you. This is not surprising as these ideas are so terrifying when you are in the middle of them. Now you know that there is another possible way of understanding your experiences, i.e. that the problem is not dangerous sensations but the *belief* that they are dangerous. The next step is to consider what you know about the world and how it fits with this alternative perspective, and what information you need to gather in order to feel more confident about it.

An extremely helpful tool to work out an alternative belief is a way of summarising your thinking and what you do, called Theory A vs. Theory B. This works for many anxiety problems. See what this looks like for Amana and Nuwa:

Amana's Theory A / Theory B	
Theory A	**Theory B**
The problem is I am physically unwell with catastrophically high blood pressure and I'm going to die, and my baby will die	The problem is I have become *preoccupied* with the feelings in my body and I have *worried* about these feelings being dangerous and meaning that something bad is happening to me and my baby. The more I have avoided anything that changes my breathing or makes my heart rate go up, the more I have worried about this. I'm now feeling miserable and scared most of the time
Evidence	

Amana's Theory A / Theory B	
No evidence of any problems with my blood pressure or other health issues	I have been told by health professionals that I am well, and that the baby is well

When I have been alone and just thinking about what my body is doing, I have had more panic attacks – thinking about bad things happening can cause panic but cannot cause pre-eclampsia (otherwise the pregnancy advice would be 'don't think about pre-eclampsia'!)

My friends have had some scary experiences, including being rushed to hospital, so it's not surprising I've been focused on bad things happening – rather than remembering all the other mothers out there who don't have medical emergencies |
| **What I need to do if this is true** | |
| Avoid any activity or movement that increases my heart rate

Monitor myself and the baby constantly for changes in any physical feeling

Ask my partner and health professionals for reassurance as often as possible

Stay in bed

Request an early delivery by C-section | Remind myself that I may have some minor risk factors for complications but so do a lot of people

Ask my partner for love and affection rather than repeated reassurance

Allow health professionals to tell me what I need to know, rather than ask them repeated questions about risks to my health

Build my confidence in my healthy body

Restore my confidence in my judgement about my health and the well-being of my baby

Go back to doing the activities that I enjoy around the house – particularly cooking

Take time to enjoy being pregnant if I can

Increase my level of physical activity to the duration and intensity of exercise recommended at this stage in pregnancy

Practise letting anxiety come and go |

Amana's Theory A / Theory B	
What does this say about the future	
My life will be extremely restricted and lonely I'll be dead	I'm going to be a kind caring mother to my baby I'll be less frightened by any unexpected physical sensations after birth

Nuwa's Theory A / Theory B	
Theory A	**Theory B**
The problem is I am going mad	The problem is I felt disoriented when I came home from hospital, because I was intensely sleep deprived and physically wrecked, and I'd been away from home for a week unexpectedly. I thought these weird feelings meant I was going 'mad', and it's not surprising that I had a massive panic attack. I didn't want to have another horrible panic attack and I continued to worry that I was going mad, and I tried really hard to avoid feeling anything intense. I believed I needed other people around to make sure nothing bad happened to the baby. I realise now that everything I did to try to make myself feel 'safe' actually made me feel more anxious.
Evidence	
None	At the times when I have been completely immersed in looking after my baby (like dealing with a massive nappy poo leakage), I haven't thought about feeling spaced out or going mad I have learned that feelings of disorientation or unreality are common and harmless feelings (especially when exhausted)

Nuwa's Theory A / Theory B	
What I need to do if this is true	
Never be alone with the baby Avoid mirrors or anything that could give me the unreal feeling Look up mental health diagnoses online and check whether the symptoms fit with my experiences Employ full-time childcare and go back to work Get myself admitted to a psychiatric hospital?	Look after my baby on my own Practise letting feelings of unreality or weirdness come and go Look in the mirror as often and for as long as I used to Practise letting feelings of anxiety come and go Tell a few close friends how bad I felt and how being on my own and isolating myself has made me feel worse Try out some of the things I planned to do with my baby – go to baby yoga, go to the park Keep to my plan to have extended maternity leave and part-time work
What does this say about the future	
I will miss out on bringing up my baby I will have to go into hospital as a long-term patient	I will go out and do things I want to do I can plan another pregnancy

Yes but … How Do I Know It's an Anxiety Problem Rather Than a Real Problem With My Health?

You might be thinking 'yes but … how can I be sure that it is an anxiety problem not an actual problem with my health?' Consider some of the things you have done to try to feel better, such as asking for reassurance, from friends or family, or medical professionals – has that actually worked? Do you feel better? The 're' bit of reassurance is the giveaway – if it worked, you wouldn't have to ask for it over and over again. What about avoiding going out, or restricting your activities – has that made you feel better? Or have you noticed that you are more focused on your body, and feeling more anxious and possibly miserable?

It is understandable that you might be thinking 'better safe than sorry' and that it is 'a small price to pay' to give up on some aspects of your life rather than 'take the risk' to your health. If you had an *actual* health problem, that would be a reasonable and appropriate decision. As you have an anxiety or worry problem, that decision to avoid certain aspects of parenting or to do things to prevent the perceived risk come at a cost.

Amana thought through the costs and the benefits of actively working to get rid of her problem with panic, versus not changing:

	Stay as I am – not change anything	Change – break free from my panic problem
Benefits	Maybe I am protecting myself and my baby from a health problem (but no-one else thinks so)	Enjoy (aspects of) my pregnancy Be healthy Enjoy usual activities Plan for the future
Costs	Restricted life – will probably get worse Deteriorating physical health from lack of exercise Feeling miserable and isolated	Accepting some uncertainty Tolerating some anxiety

Try drawing out the cost and benefits for you:

	Stay as I am – not change anything	Change – break free from my panic problem
Benefits		
Costs		

OVER TO YOU
Reset Your Goals: What Are You Working Towards?

Nuwa had been independent and determined before she had the panic attacks. She thought about what she really wanted to be doing. Writing down her goals gave her the courage to start making changes and overcome her problem with panic:

Questions to ask myself	My goals	How hard is this for me now 0 = not able to do 10 = complete success
What do I want to be doing in the next few weeks?	1. Being with my baby on my own	5
	2. Going to the park with my baby	4
	3. Looking in the mirror like I used to – put on some make-up	1
What do I want to be doing in the next few months?	1. Going on a long train journey to go on holiday	0
	2. Have a 'welcome to the world' party for my baby with 30+ guests	1
	3. Join a baby yoga group	2
What do I want to be doing by this time next year?	1. Planning another pregnancy	1
	2. Moving house	1
	3. Looking for a new job	2

Keeping these goals in mind reminded her that putting up with some anxiety and even some panic in the short term was worth it, so that she could go back to living her life freely.

You now have an understanding of how panic works for you. Remind yourself why you are prepared to tackle this problem and what you can claim back if you get rid of panic – don't get caught up in thinking about how you overcome the panic, think about what it will be like when it is no longer a problem. It's fine to take this in steps – any changes will help move you towards recovery.

Questions to ask myself	My goals	
		How hard is this for me now 0 = not able to do 10 = complete success
What do I want to be doing in the next few weeks?		
What do I want to be doing in the next few months?		
What do I want to be doing by this time next year?		

Don't worry if you can't think of many goals – having one or two specific goals will still help you to 'keep your eyes on the prize'.

Moving Forward: Tackling Your Anxiety-related Thinking

It is really important to test things in an active way, and not when you are in the middle of an unexpected panic attack. Putting the theory into practice will really help you learn – it's a bit like the importance of playing the guitar rather than just studying the theory.

> Amana was terrified of any change in her breathing or heart rate. She sat on her bed for most of the day, avoiding using the stairs and never going outside. Her midwives had urged her to be active and that she had nothing to worry about, but every time she tried to move around more, she noticed a change in her body such as breathlessness or a racing heart, and was terrified that this meant she was going to die.

Amana decided to experiment with deliberately changing her breathing, to build up her belief in her Theory B – that the changes in her body were normal, and that the problem was that she was over-focused on them and worrying about them. This is in contrast to Theory A – that the physical feelings are a sign of danger. She started off doing an everyday ordinary activity – walking around her home. She then deliberately altered her breathing to find out what actually happened:

Complete before the experiment		Complete after the experiment		
Planned experiment	My specific predictions and how much I believe them	Did my predictions come true?	What are my conclusions?	Does this fit best with Theory A or Theory B?
Get up and walk around my home for 10 minutes without stopping or asking for reassurance	My breathing will be out of control and will stop (100%) My heart will race (100%) and I will have a heart attack (20%) I will become very unwell requiring emergency medical assistance (80%)	My breathing was fast and irregular but evened out after a few minutes, and did not stop (0%) My heart did race but I did not have a heart attack (0%) I did not become unwell (0%)	When I left my breathing and heart rate alone, it sorted itself out (like it always has done in the past – when I used to go to exercise classes I would breathe hard and fast but then my breathing and heart rate would return to normal without me trying to do anything about it)	Fits better with Theory B – that I have become preoccupied with the feelings in my body and I have worried about these feelings being dangerous – but actually this is worry / anxiety / in my thinking, rather than an actual threat to my physical health

Complete before the experiment		Complete after the experiment		
Planned experiment	My specific predictions and how much I believe them	Did my predictions come true?	What are my conclusions?	Does this fit best with Theory A or Theory B?
Make my breathing faster and shallower by breathing through a straw (to make breathing harder) for 60 seconds without trying to adjust my breathing afterwards	My breathing will stop and I'll suffocate (50%)	My breathing was fast whilst I was breathing through the straw, then returned to normal within a minute of stopping breathing through the straw (0%)	I deliberately put my breathing under pressure and even though I felt quite anxious, nothing bad happened to me	
	I will feel extremely anxious (10/10 anxiety for at least two hours) (100%)	I felt 9/10 anxious but for a few minutes, then it went down to 2–3/10 for another 10–20 minutes (0%)		
	I will have a panic attack (100%)	I felt strange but I did not panic (0%)		

Yes but … Is It Safe to Overbreathe in Pregnancy?

We always tailor our planned experiments and activities to fit with the situation a person is in. We wouldn't advise a heavily pregnant woman to run on the spot for five minutes, which we might do in other circumstances. The idea of the experiment is to approach the sensations that you have been avoiding, and it is likely that in pregnancy you will need to do less in order to bring them on.

What might have stopped Amana finding out that she could have all sorts of changes in her breathing and nothing bad happened? If she had started breathing into a paper bag, or asked for reassurance, she would not have been able to make the same conclusions. As outlined in the 'what keeps the processes going' table, doing anything that 'buys into' the idea that something bad is going to happen, stops you from finding out what happens if you just keep going. Start where you can, but try and drop your safety-seeking behaviours.

Nuwa is worried about different physical sensations and has a different belief to test out:

Panic attacks can bring up lots of odd sensations that you can test out in exactly the way described above. Below are some more examples.

Feared sensation	Possible experiments
Racing heart	Walk up and down stairs
Short of breath	Breathe in and out more quickly Breathe through a straw Hold breath for 15 seconds
Visual disturbance	Look up 'moving optical illusions' on the Internet
Feeling hot	Sit near a radiator for 5 minutes

Complete before the experiment		Complete after the experiment		
Planned behavioural experiment	My specific predictions and how much I believe them	Did my predictions come true?	What are my conclusions?	Does this fit best with Theory A or Theory B?
Finding out about whether other people have feelings of weirdness and what they think about what I experience – survey of friends asking 'do you ever feel really spaced out and like you are not really there'	No-one else will experience these feelings (80%) (I have read online that some people do, but I'm not sure it's quite the same or as dangerous)	I asked five people: Two other people had felt very spaced out and weird during or after childbirth, including one friend who thought that all her possessions looked so odd that she even doubted they were her own, and had a weird feeling that she had twins when she did not.	Other people's thinking was a lot weirder than I anticipated No-one thought that it was anything bad or dangerous when I told them I felt so unreal (5% belief that no-one will have these feelings and that everyone will think it is really strange)	Fits better with Theory B – that by focusing on these feelings and avoiding situations when I bring them on, I have got stuck with the idea that the weird sensations mean something bad, and that I shouldn't be left on my own looking after my baby
'I had a really strong feeling of unreality when I came home from hospital – what do you think was going on?'	Everyone will think it is really strange that I had these feelings (90%)	Nobody thought it was strange, people said 'not that surprising if you had just had that week in hospital and the difficult birth' 'I feel weird most of the time as I'm so desperate for sleep!'		

Complete before the experiment		Complete after the experiment		
Planned behavioural experiment	**My specific predictions and how much I believe them**	**Did my predictions come true?**	**What are my conclusions?**	**Does this fit best with Theory A or Theory B?**
Looking in the mirror for five minutes non-stop to bring on the unreal feeling	I will feel unreal (100%) And I will lose control, e.g. start screaming (50%)	I did feel unreal (100%) I did not lose control (0%) I started thinking of other things	Looking at myself in the mirror for a long time does make me feel weird, but that doesn't mean that anything bad is going on	
Comparing a day of checking online for symptoms of mental ill health versus a day of not checking	Checking for symptoms of serious mental illness makes me feel less anxious (50%) Not checking will make me feel more anxious (95%)	On the day I checked throughout the day, I felt *more anxious*, compared to the day when I did not (0%)	I thought checking online was helping me but I realise it was making me worse	This is evidence against Theory A This helps build up evidence for Theory B, as it shows that when I do not react to the physical sensations, I feel less anxious

Moving Forward: What Can You Do to Break Free from Panic?

If you are not sure where to start with your own behavioural experiments, then think about what you are not doing / what you are avoiding, and pick one of those things. Plan doing it 'normally' without taking precautions.

What's the worst thing that could happen – what does Theory A say?

How does the world really work – what does Theory B say?

Complete before the experiment		Complete after the experiment		
Planned behavioural experiment	My specific predictions and how much I believe them	Did my predictions come true?	What are my conclusions?	Does this fit best with Theory A or Theory B?

Don't Stop There: Beating Panic Attacks in the Long Term

Amana felt happy for the first time in a while, and was confidently moving around her home and enjoying cooking again. However, she still had an idea at the back of her mind that her blood pressure would be a problem, and still felt cautious about raising her heart rate. She agreed to do a behavioural experiment with another pregnant friend who knew that Amana had lost her confidence in physical activity and had been feeling anxious. They walked up and down the stairs continually for five minutes, which they both found to be hard work. They both experienced their hearts pounding and feeling out of breath. They also made each other laugh by talking about all the different bits of their bodies that had changed since pregnancy, and joking about how long they could last before one of them needed the loo. Amana was able to do this again, alone, and repeated it a few times to make sure that she was overcoming this last bit of avoidance.

It's understandable to want to 'quit while I'm ahead' after you have made some progress with overcoming panic. It is important to keep going until you have worked on all the different things that keep the problem going – anything that you are avoiding, or do differently because of your fears that something is going wrong with your body. If you are wondering if it's worth it, go back to your list of goals and remind yourself what you are working towards. At the end of the book (Chapter 10), we have a 'blueprint' to record the key ideas and progress you have made.

To Sum Up

- A panic attack is a sudden rush of intense fear and physical sensations. They can often feel like they strike without warning
- Physical sensations in your body fluctuate and change, and you may be very 'tuned in' to noticing these changes, especially when you are pregnant and after childbirth
- Noticing physical changes in your body and interpreting these sensations as dangerous when they are not, leads to extreme and terrifying anxiety and panic
- Significant anxiety about your health can happen when you believe the physical symptoms you experience mean that you are unwell with a serious physical illness such as cancer (even though you have been checked out)

- Paying very close attention to your physical feelings, trying to do things to reduce the physical feelings, or avoiding situations or activities for fear of having a panic attack, can make the problem worse
- Allowing physical feelings to come and go, and finding out that anxiety will pass, will help you get back to 'normal' life
- Reducing physical checking and reassurance seeking will help you be less worried about your health

6

Feeling Anxious Around Other People

In this chapter you will learn:

➤ What social anxiety is and why it can be very difficult in the perinatal period

➤ How particular thoughts, behaviours and self-focused attention can keep it going

➤ How to make changes to feel more confident around others

➤ How to be less hard on your own performance in various situations

---

It is really common to feel self-conscious on occasion around others, worrying that people might be thinking badly of you or noticing that you are anxious. For some people, this is a regular occurrence that happens in almost any social situation or repeatedly in particular situations such as being in a group of people, being at work and so on. They may find themselves worrying about what it will be like before going, effortfully enduring it whilst there, taking measures to reduce the likelihood of others thinking badly of them, and thinking about it a great deal afterwards to evaluate how they came across. It might feel easier to avoid these situations in the first place. These are all very well-known features of social anxiety.

You may find that social interactions trigger severe anxiety and a strong sense that people will notice this and judge you for it. Examples would be a fear of saying the wrong thing in a group with other mums, that your baby may cry and somehow show that you are not competent, or feeling like you may seem anxious or come across badly in a conversation with a health professional.

You may always have been affected by this problem, or maybe it has just started to bother you more as you journey into motherhood – whatever your situation, the techniques we describe here can help you to get away from this horrible feeling of intense self-consciousness and anxiety and refocus on enjoying time with your baby and other people. Like most anxiety problems, there is no one clear cause of social anxiety, but it makes sense that the huge changes in life that come about with pregnancy and becoming a parent may amplify an existing self-consciousness, or could unexpectedly provoke this specific anxiety when you find yourself in new and very unfamiliar situations, and having to interact with a lot of different people.

How Being Pregnant or a New Parent Can Be Difficult if You Are Anxious Around Other People

If you have been used to being a bit of a 'wallflower' (staying in the background when in the company of others), that is often no longer possible in pregnancy or after birth. Pregnancy and having a new baby draw attention to you from people you know and people you have never met. In the later stages of pregnancy, you naturally take up more space and move more slowly, so there is more to notice. Once your baby is here, they may well attract attention even if you don't want it. For some people, the extra attention is enjoyable or at least tolerable, but even a trip to the shops can be extremely unpleasant and upsetting if being the focus of attention is a problem for you. Loved ones or sometimes even strangers might offer you advice or comments on your pregnancy and parenting that may be well-meant but just end up making you feel self-conscious or judged.

For example, you may feel very self-conscious about the sound of your baby crying. If you are anxious, you may think that everyone is looking at you and thinking badly of you. In reality that is very seldom the case. Your baby crying or being distressed can elicit strong emotional and physical responses – you may notice yourself feeling very anxious, panicky and you may produce breast milk if you hear any baby cry. However, even though your baby's cry is designed to attract *your* attention, other people may not even notice it. If you walk out into a crowded area and see a baby crying, the parent or carer may be very focused on the baby, but other people are unlikely to pay much attention, if any at all. There is a difference between how *you* experience a situation like this and how others do. As you read this chapter, you will find out more about how this feeling of self-consciousness is maintained and learn to use this information to combat the associated anxiety.

OVER TO YOU

Is Anxiety in Situations with Other People a Problem for You?

What social situations are difficult for you (or do you anticipate might be difficult after your baby is born)?

What do you worry might happen? Are there specific things you fear you or your baby might say or do that you think others would notice and judge negatively?

How do you think people would judge you? What do you worry this says about you?

How does your anxiety in situations with other people affect you? What does it stop you from doing, or what does it make more difficult?

Let's consider some examples of how this problem works:

Social Anxiety in Pregnancy

Ziva

Ziva was pregnant for the first time. She worked in a high-pressure City job. She enjoyed the work when she was on her own for long periods analysing data and programming.

She had always struggled with anxiety in meetings, dreading having to speak up – she often worried that people would think she was unintelligent, silly or a fraud. She had heard colleagues criticise each other for making errors, both face-to-face and in private. A recent promotion resulted in the requirement to attend more meetings and an expectation of speaking up more.

Becoming pregnant raised Ziva's anxiety, as there were very few women in her organisation and none in a senior role. She was congratulated by her colleagues but she feared that pregnancy and requesting maternity leave was another reason for them to consider her weak and incompetent. When she felt hot and flushed due to pregnancy, she hated that this drew attention to her at work and worried that her colleagues would think that she was not capable of doing her job.

Ziva knew that when she was on maternity leave, she would need – and want – to talk to other new parents, and already started to worry about what it would be like in parent and baby groups when speaking to people she didn't know very well. She could already picture herself in these settings, looking like she didn't know what she was doing, red-faced and tearful.

In her birth preparation classes, she had stayed on the sidelines, rehearsed what she would say, and made excuses to go as soon as possible at the end of the session. When the birth preparation group set up a messaging group, she would scrutinise the replies to her messages, anticipating negative or dismissive comments from others, or that her messages would be ignored.

Social Anxiety Postnatally

Kali

Kali's baby suffered with colic, which meant he had frequent bouts of intense and inconsolable crying. Kali found the crying extremely hard to cope with. Nothing she tried seemed to help him settle. She felt helpless and sad that she wasn't able to enjoy her baby in the way she hoped.

Other mums in her antenatal group had been sharing pictures and stories of their happy trips out with their new baby but Kali was struggling to leave the house. The thought of being in public with a screaming baby made her feel too anxious, so she avoided going out with him as much as possible. If she did have to go out, she felt extremely tense and on edge. Her heart would race and she would feel a huge sense of dread. She would make sure she kept a close eye out for any signs her baby was becoming upset and make a swift exit home if he did start to cry.

Staying as close to home as possible meant she could get back quickly if she needed to. If he was crying, she would feel intensely self-conscious, as if all eyes were on her. She would feel hot, embarrassed and trembly and usually start to cry. She had an image in her head of looking scared, tearful and flushed whilst she held her screaming baby frozen to the spot. His crying was so loud she was convinced it stopped people in their tracks, that they would notice how panicked she was and think 'what a clueless mum! Why isn't she helping her baby?' She worried they would laugh about it with other people for days to come.

In Kali's mind, good mothers didn't have crying babies like hers. She would do her best to avoid eye contact or conversations in shops, for fear people would see how anxious she was or that talking to anyone might delay her long enough that he would start to cry. Meeting up with other friends and their babies felt impossible, as everyone else's baby seemed so settled and calm (which made her feel like a failure) and Kali simply couldn't relax or concentrate on what other people were saying. This left her feeling lonely. When alone, she would spend long periods of time going over what had happened when she was out, confirming her fears that she had come across to others as unable to calm her baby or cope with the situation.

What Keeps You Stuck in Social Anxiety: Factors in the Present

Feeling extremely self-conscious and anxious leads to some understandable reactions. You might become aware of physical sensations such as feeling hot and sweaty, which feel very intense and noticeable. You might also be trying to limit or 'manage' the social situation in some way or avoid these situations altogether. However, not seeing anyone ever is not a realistic or healthy option when you are pregnant or a new parent. There will be various routine clinical appointments to attend, you will want to see people you care about and introduce them to your baby, and your baby will need to explore new places and meet new people.

Like all other anxiety difficulties, some ways of thinking and behaving that you do with the intention to make yourself feel better actually keep anxiety going. We will look at ways to break out of these ways of thinking and behaving, and how you can work towards being more comfortable and less self-conscious in social situations.

Getting Drawn into the Feeling of Anxiety 'How I Feel Is How I Look'

We don't experience ourselves from the outside. When you are feeling very anxious, it feels very easy to believe that everyone is noticing your anxiety and judging you, because the feelings are so intense. This can be compounded if you start remembering other times when you felt embarrassed, or when something humiliating or shameful happened. These images and memories start to interfere with your thinking and draw you further into the feeling of anxiety – your fears start to *feel* like reality, e.g. that people are looking at you, they have noticed something embarrassing you said or did and are now thinking negatively about you.

Like Kali, you might worry that they are then going to ponder it for days and share your embarrassing anecdote with all their friends. In reality, it is more likely that they haven't noticed anything and are simply minding their own business. Even if they did notice, it's very unlikely that they will be judgemental. They might be more worried about you if you are avoiding meeting up. However, this information about how the world really works can get lost when you feel very anxious.

For Kali, she had an image in her head of looking scared, tearful and flushed whilst she held her screaming baby, frozen to the spot. For Ziva, she pictured herself looking like she didn't know what she was doing, red-faced and tearful. Both believed that this image was exactly what was seen by other people.

Beliefs About Being Judged

Ziva had a longstanding belief that she would be judged by others, reinforced by her experiences at work. She thought about being in the antenatal class, and wrote down what was going on in her thinking:

Questions to ask myself	
What images or thoughts come to mind?	Image of looking anxious and tearful with a bright red face
What's so bad about having this thought?	I look foolish and incompetent, like I can't hold it together
What makes it hard to ignore or dismiss?	Other people do judge – I know this as my colleagues at work talk about people behind their backs
What does the fact you are having these thoughts mean about you?	I'm not as good as everyone else
What's the worst thing about this thought?	I'll be criticised and ridiculed by others
What's the very worst thing about this?	I will be rejected and alone

It was difficult for her to step away from this idea, despite knowing that antenatal classes were not the same as work, and that the people seemed genuine and kind, and wanted to get to know her.

KEY IDEA

When you feel anxious in social situations, you may have a negative image of how you appear to others, and that they will judge you based on how you look and come across.

OVER TO YOU
What Are You Thinking when You Feel Anxious?

Think of the last time that you felt extremely anxious around others – what was going through your mind? Can you capture any of the thoughts or images that were going through your head? If this is too difficult to remember, then imagine being in a social situation and see what comes into your head. Remember, you do not have to find an answer for all of these questions – they are prompts to get you thinking about your thinking. Just do as much as you can.

What thoughts or images come to mind? What's so bad about having this thought? What makes it hard to ignore or dismiss? What does the fact you are having these thoughts mean about you? What's the worst thing about this thought? What's the very worst thing about this?	

Self-focused Attention

We all have a finite amount of attention that we can pay to ourselves and to others and the environment around us, so we focus on the things that seem most important. When we are self-conscious, as the term suggests, most of our attention is usually focused inward onto ourselves and it becomes increasingly difficult to be aware of what is happening around us. Focusing in on yourself makes sense if you believe that you really are at risk of being criticised or judged – you are trying to protect yourself from this 'social threat'. If you have noticed your attention going inwards when you feel anxious in social situations, don't be hard on yourself – it's your brain trying to keep you safe by narrowing your focus. This is part of our 'fight or flight' response (see Chapter 1). Unfortunately, this has the effect of keeping your anxiety in social situations going, as:

1. you miss out on the opportunity to see what is actually going on around you
2. you find it harder to concentrate on the task in hand (e.g. the conversation), and
3. you end up with magnified feelings of self-consciousness as attention is like a zoom lens

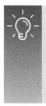 **KEY IDEA**

When you are socially anxious your attention is focused on yourself and how you are coming across rather than on the situation as a whole.

Things You Do to Manage the Perceived Threat: Safety-seeking Behaviours

If you believe you are under threat of negative judgement or ridicule by others, then it makes sense to try to make yourself feel safer. You might do this in advance of social situations by rehearsing what you are going to say, or sticking to certain topics during conversations, or making excuses to arrive late or leave early. In CBT we call all these physical or mental actions 'safety-seeking behaviours', and if you have read other chapters, you will see how safety-seeking behaviours map onto the specific fear that you experience. Whilst these behaviours are designed to make you feel safer or better, they usually draw you back into the idea that something bad is happening or about to happen.

Ziva was offered a glass of water during the antenatal class. She didn't want to take it as she feared that people would see her hands shaking, but the session had included advice on staying hydrated so if she didn't take it, she feared the other group members would ask her questions or judge her. She felt stuck between a rock and a hard place. She took the drink but held it very tightly to try to control shaking. She focused on the glass and whether it was shaking, and had a horrible image of her hands uncontrollably trembling, and found it difficult to follow the rest of the conversation, going blank when people asked her questions as she hadn't been listening. Ziva felt more self-conscious, then got more hot, shaky and upset, then even more focused on herself, cranking up her self-consciousness even more.

Ziva's efforts to try to feel more in control of her anxiety made her feel *more* self-conscious, and made her less engaged in the group discussion, and actually drew more attention to herself as she struggled to answer the questions. The tighter she held the glass, the more likely she was to actually tremble.

When Ziva got home, she replayed the situation in her head, and felt convinced that everyone else in the group thought she was foolish; she considered whether to drop out of the classes.

Ziva's 'post-match analysis' or 'post mortem' of what happened made her feel worse, as she could only replay her experience of feeling self-conscious. She was unable to bring in any other information about what actually happened, as she had not been aware of it at the time.

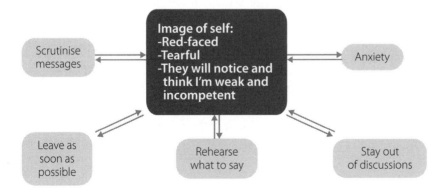

Here are some other examples:

What I do when feeling self-conscious	What is the unintended consequence?
I focus on my baby to avoid attention on myself	Stops me from finding out that others are not looking at me. Feeds into my self-consciousness about what I'm doing
I look at my baby to avoid eye contact with others	Stops me seeing that others are not judging me. Stops me connecting with other people properly
Focus attention on myself and how anxious I feel and how I think I look to others	Exaggerates my feelings of anxiety. Makes me feel like it is really noticeable
I avoid feeding my baby in front of others	Stops me finding out that I can do this and that others don't pay as much attention as I fear
If my baby is upset, I will leave the social situation	Stops me finding out I can cope with this
I keep the topic of conversation on the baby	Reinforces the idea that I'm not interesting and have nothing in common with people. Can be a bit unnatural
I avoid speaking to other parents I don't know well	People might think I'm unfriendly

Safety behaviours like these can actually make things worse as they stop you being yourself in social situations.

KEY IDEA

You do things to try to avoid the situation, or to try to hide yourself or your anxiety in the situation, and may think about it for a long time afterwards – all of which get in the way of you finding out 'how the world really works'.

OVER TO YOU
How Do You 'Manage' Social Anxiety?

Do you do anything in social situations to try to draw attention away from yourself, or to control the way you appear to others, or do anything in advance to prepare, or anything afterwards to 'analyse' the situation? What are the unintended consequences of these behaviours?

OVER TO YOU
What Are Your Goals? What Do You Want to Be Doing When You Feel More at Ease in Social Situations?

Have a think about what you want to be doing when you feel more at ease in social situations – there are no rules for what you do or don't do, and it doesn't have to include the same things as other people you know. Maybe parent and baby singing groups are not for you but joining an exercise class would work for you. Try to get away from any 'I should be doing … ', as this might get you stuck in some self-criticism. Right now, it might be enough to aim for getting out of the house and going for a walk around the block.

Kali thought about what she really wanted to be doing. Writing down her goals gave her the courage to start making changes and overcome her difficulties in social situations:

> **What do I want to be doing in the next few weeks?**
> Going out at least once a day with my baby
> Go to the local park and café with my friend
> **What do I want to be doing in the next few months?**
> Take my baby into work to meet my colleagues
> Take up spontaneous offers to go out and meet people
> **What do I want to be doing by this time next year?**
> Go to settling-in days at the nursery
> Go on a camping holiday

Keeping these goals in mind reminded her that putting up with some anxiety was worth it, so that she could enjoy her time with her baby, and be genuinely free to choose what she did or didn't do with other people.

You now have an understanding of how anxiety works for you. Remind yourself why you are prepared to tackle this problem:

	How hard is this for me now 1 = not hard, I can do it 10 = impossible
What do I want to be doing in the next few weeks?	
What do I want to be doing in the next few months?	
What do I want to be doing by this time next year?	

Don't worry if you can't think of many goals; having one or two specific goals will still help you to keep focused on what you need to do.

Moving Forward: Tackling Your Anxiety-related Thinking in Social Situations

What We Know Helps with Overcoming Anxiety in Social Situations

CBT has been shown to be a very effective treatment for this problem. In CBT we work on your anxiety-related thinking to highlight the difference between feeling anxious and looking anxious, and what happens when you shift your focus to the situation around you, rather than what's going on in your head, and what happens when you don't take extra precautions.

Comparing Image and Reality: 'People Will Notice Me Looking Anxious'

Ziva believed that other people noticed her getting hot and uncomfortable when she was in her birth preparation class and had a vivid image in her head of what she looked like – red and flustered, with a despairing look on her face. She agreed with her partner that they would take a picture of her during the antenatal class, so that she could see what she really looked like. She worried that this was going to be difficult to do in the class, and couldn't bring herself to do it for a couple of weeks. When she was courageous enough to try it, to her surprise the other group members jumped at the chance to have a photo taken as a memento, and it all happened really quickly. When she looked at the photo afterwards, she felt herself zooming in on her face to check for redness or looking despairing. When she looked at it objectively, she saw that she was no more red or sweaty than others with a similar skin tone, and she looked surprised but happy in the photo. She kept the photo stuck on her fridge to remind her that the image in her head of herself looking very anxious is not what others actually see, and to remind her that going to the antenatal classes was very difficult at the time, but worth it.

You might find it difficult to get 'objective' information about what you look like and the idea of staging a photo might be too much to consider. The main idea to remember with this is that what you see in your head is an exaggeration and is built on feeling anxious and self-conscious. You might not think you look amazing or completely poised, but the idea is that there will be a difference between the image in your head, and what other people see. Even if you get a bit of shift towards remembering this, it will help you to feel less anxious.

Another idea to try is to over-emphasise what you believe people notice – if you think your hands shake, deliberately shake them more and see what happens. Slosh your drink on the carpet and see what people do or say.

Finally, even if you are a bit red, or people do notice some shaking, so what? Does this mean you shouldn't be allowed to live your life freely and enjoy time out and about? Is that a standard you would apply to others? We will look at an example of how to challenge your thinking below.

Testing Out Your Anxiety-related Thinking: What Do Other People Really Think?

Kali believed that other mothers thought that she was 'clueless' and that she was unable to help her baby, and that they would laugh at her or even be angry with her.

It was too difficult for Kali to ask other people about this, so she messaged a small group of friends that she didn't see often, but to whom she still felt close. She described the scene she played over and over in her head, *'I was out last week with the baby and he screamed his head off the whole time, I felt like a terrible mum and that everyone else was doing a better job – I've not been out since [sad face].'*

She was nervous sending the message as she didn't want to admit that she was finding things difficult, as this felt like it might confirm her thinking that she was a failure. She predicted that her friends would not answer, or would send messages that dismissed her concerns, such as 'get over it, just get on with it,' or that showed their shock or disapproval, 'he cried all the time, can't you soothe him?'.

However, all her friends responded with kind messages, 'what a rubbish day, it's such hard work, I bet you are doing a great job,' 'I bet all the other mums there were really feeling for you,' 'I wish I'd been there to give you a hand – it's so relentless, I bet you need a breather.' One friend didn't reply for a couple of days, which made Kali doubt herself more, but then did reply saying 'sorry not to get back to you, I'm feeling really rough myself as baby not sleeping – been in tears most of the last few days – thank goodness my sister is coming to stay as I'm at my wits end – so good to hear from you and really want to see you soon.'

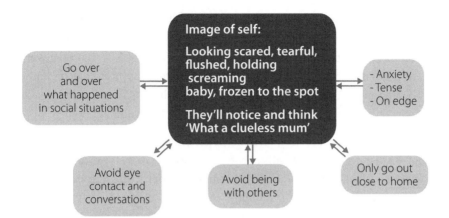

Kali was able to take on board that her friends cared about her, thought well of her and could empathise with her. By being honest with her friends, she learned about their difficulties, and she was able to send her friend supportive and caring messages in return. She found it helpful to go back to their messages when she was feeling anxious, as the messages reminded her that feeling this way is not proof of coming across badly to others.

However, the idea that the other mothers were 'feeling for her' rather than judging her still didn't feel that believable, so Kali arranged to go out with a friend who had a slightly older baby who also was prone to loud crying and was difficult to soothe. When her friend's baby cried very loudly and threw his toys, Kali very deliberately paid attention to the other parents in the park. She noticed that some other parents immediately turned and looked, but then quickly went back to their own child. Some parents gave sympathetic looks. Two parents picked up the toys and made kind remarks to her friend. Kali was surprised by their reactions and learned several things:

- When she directed her attention on others rather than being stuck in her own thinking, she noticed that people were not looking at her friend or making disapproving noises or faces
- People did not judge
- People helped

Kali then stayed in the park; after a short while her baby cried very loudly. Whilst she comforted the baby, she actively looked / directed her attention at others. She noticed that other parents were absorbed with their own babies, and rarely looked in her direction. A well-dressed and calm-looking parent came up to her and Kali had a rush of fear that they were going to say that she was doing a bad job – in fact they asked if she had a size 3 nappy as they had run out. Kali was delighted to help a stranger and amazed that someone who looked so 'in control' needed her help.

When it was time to leave, another mum offered to get her buggy sorted out for her whilst Kali continued to comfort her baby, and did this in a 'matter of fact' way, which slightly unnerved her. Once the other mum had finished sorting out the buggy, she smiled and said she was always a bit nervous unfolding other people's buggies in case she couldn't do it, and made a funny remark about folding and unfolding buggies and looking after babies being a great deal harder than being at work. Kali was surprised to hear that the other mother was nervous.

Kali realised that she had rarely spent enough time in a situation to find out what actually happened when things were going 'wrong'. When she deliberately stayed in a situation and directed her attention away from her own self-consciousness and on to the scene around her, what actually happened is that she experienced a sense of solidarity and support from the other parents, with sympathetic and helpful reactions.

Kali made a deal with herself to go out every day, even if she felt anxious, and even if her baby was having an unsettled day. She started to see familiar faces and feel more confident to be out and about, and she noticed what her baby particularly enjoyed about being out – the bright lights in the café, the noise of a nearby school playground, and the smell of the bakery that they often stopped in. She felt proud of herself for building up a new way of being.

OVER TO YOU
Testing Things Out

Can you plan to do something that would test out your ideas about other people?

Using the table below will help you stick to the task. Here is what Kali tested out:

What am I testing out?		What did I find out?	
My belief that other parents think I am clueless and will judge me as incompetent			
My plan	**My specific predictions and how much I believe them (%)**	**Did my predictions come true?**	**What are my conclusions? What does this tell me about how the world really works?**
Go to the park when it is busy and stay there when the baby is crying, and deliberately look at other people to see what they are doing	Other parents will make disapproving faces (rolling their eyes, frowning) and noises (tutting, muttering under their breath) (95%) Other parents will come over to me and criticise me (40%)	No Nobody disapproved of me Hardly anyone looked at me	Even when I am feeling anxious and self-conscious, and even when the baby is crying loudly, other people are not judging me or criticising me, or giving me any actual indication that they think I am clueless Other people helped me and asked for my help – they must think I'm at least a bit competent!

Try and use the table below:

What am I testing out?		What did I find out?	
My plan	**My specific predictions and how much I believe them**	**Did my predictions come true?**	**What are my conclusions? What does this tell me about how the world really works?**

Moving Forward: Building Confidence Gradually

Ziva found conversations with smaller groups of people easier. She made a social date with another parent from the birth preparation group and tried not to rehearse or prepare for the conversation:

What am I testing out?			
My plan	My specific predictions and how much I believe them (%)	Did my predictions come true?	What are my conclusions? What does this tell me about how the world really works?
Meet a friend Not prepare anything beforehand	I won't be able to think of anything to say (100%) Unless I prepare in advance, I will come across really badly and they will leave (95%) and make excuses so that they never have to meet with me again (100%)	No She didn't leave and in fact we stayed out for longer than we both expected. It turned out we had loads in common and it was easy to talk Occasionally there was a pause in conversation and I felt uneasy, but we got talking again quickly each time	I suppose no conversation goes completely perfectly I still felt anxious and worried that I was coming across badly, but some of the time I was just enjoying the conversation

Ziva built on what she learned by agreeing to a larger gathering from the group. She felt very anxious at the beginning and tried to stay out of the conversation, but remembered what she had learned from talking to her friend individually and told everyone in the group some of the things they had in common. This sparked an interesting conversation and Ziva was able to join in.

You will need to do things more than once to start feeling better. Plan to repeat the same kind of task, or work out a way to make it more challenging each time.

Yes but … What if They Really Are Judging Me?

What if Ziva had been out with a group of friends and they had all left before her, some without saying goodbye? In these ambiguous situations, we need to look out for 'mind reading' – if Ziva had thought 'they all left because of me', can we look and see if there are any other possibilities? For example, her friends leaving as they needed to be somewhere else, feeling unwell or tired, worrying that their baby needed to get home for a nap or food, the baby had vomited and poo-ed on all its clothes and they were out of spares …

There are lots of times when we don't know for sure what people are thinking or what is behind their actions, so watch out for jumping to the conclusion that other people's actions or reactions are directly related to you and how you are coming across. No matter how much your anxiety is telling you otherwise, it is more likely that they haven't noticed anything significant about you and are not judging you. If a person really is judging you, for example they said something clearly disapproving, you might consider if this is a person whose opinion you really do value and respect. Would you say this to a friend in a similar circumstance? See the end of this chapter for dealing with criticism.

Being Hard on Yourself: Setting Impossibly High Standards

With social anxiety we can feel judged by others. It can also feel that everyone else is doing things well and better than us. Another style of thinking that can contribute to feeling anxious and low in mood is to have excessively high standards for yourself – you think that you should always come up with the absolutely best answer to any question, or that you should be getting everything 'right'. Babies definitely interfere with being able to answer any question, and frequently interfere with getting anything done, let alone getting it 'right'!

Pregnancy and having a new baby do not mix well with very high, inflexible standards, where you judge yourself harshly if you don't do things to your own exacting standards. It's a good thing to want to give your baby the best start in life, but you are making it harder to achieve this if you are being highly perfectionist, and you run the risk of feeling anxious and miserable by being too hard on yourself, or avoiding altogether some aspects of your baby's care ('if I can't do this perfectly, I'm not doing it at all'). You might have been able to be perfectionist at work, or keep your house very neat and ordered, or maintain high standards of appearance and healthy habits – in the new world you find yourself in with your pregnancy and new baby, your old rules are going to be very hard to follow.

How Perfectionism Works

Having high standards is not a problem – being driven or ambitious is not a problem. Pursuing this at all costs, and judging yourself harshly when you do not meet your own excessively high or rigid standards can be a problem. Perfectionism is described as when you find yourself judging your self-worth solely on your achievements (rather than all your qualities and interests), and when you apply a 'pass / fail' judgement on whether you have done something 'right', and with the idea that you must always get it right – no exceptions, no excuses. Roz Shafran, Sarah Egan and Tracey Wade have researched perfectionism and worked out the key problems, and how to approach them in CBT.

Perfectionism in the Postnatal Period: Anaisa

Anaisa was delighted to have her new baby. She wanted to have her first baby when she was 28, no older, no younger, and this had worked out. The birth went well and she and her baby were healthy. She had prepared the baby's room with a carefully thought through colour scheme and with decorations and toys that were designed to promote the baby's development. The first few weeks with her newborn were wonderful, and she enjoyed responding to her baby's needs and introducing her to family and friends. After another few weeks of sleepless nights, and when her partner went back to work, she started to feel very stressed about the untidy house, and that there were piles of unwashed clothes, and that she looked tired and drawn. She had some invitations to go out and meet other parents, but she often turned these down as she had some strict ideas about what things should be like when she left the house, that were becoming more impossible to achieve, such as:

The baby must always be happy and never crying.

I must always be prepared for every eventuality when we are out.

I must look calm and in control, and be well-dressed and groomed.

When her baby was asleep, she spent all her time cleaning the house. She felt annoyed with her partner for not doing enough – when they came home from work her partner was desperate to play with the baby, but she resented them for having all the fun when she was so preoccupied with laundry and housework.

We can already take a guess at what thinking is behind Anaisa's rules:

If I don't have a clean and tidy house, then people will think I'm not coping and am failing as a mother.

I should be on top of the laundry – a basic household task – if I am not, then this shows how totally useless I am.

If the baby isn't happy and is crying, then I'm not 100% meeting her needs and totally failing at motherhood.

If I don't have absolutely everything I need when I'm out, other people will judge me as completely disorganised and flaky.

If I don't look calm, collected and well-groomed, then it's a slippery slope to being constantly dishevelled and unwashed, and being a disgrace.

We can spot the all or nothing, black and white thinking, and how harshly Anaisa is evaluating herself. If she didn't perform to her high standards, she judged herself as failing – both at that specific task and overall as a person. There is nothing wrong with trying to keep yourself and your house tidy, and certainly nothing wrong with trying to be prepared in how you respond to your baby's needs. However, trying to do this to a punishingly high standard, all of the time, is impossible, and the very real danger is evaluating yourself as 'failing' when you are actually doing a fantastic job (probably in difficult circumstances). The consequence is feeling anxious, angry, guilty or sad, all of which are difficult feelings and might make you even more determined to pursue your high standards. This will come at the cost of your well-being, eating into your sleep, your sense of humour, your ability to be spontaneous, and perhaps your relationships with others.

OVER TO YOU
Do You Have Unhelpful Perfectionism?

Do you use perfectionist rules? Can you spot any thoughts or rules like this in your thinking? Think of occasions when you feel particularly anxious, and see if anything like this is driving what you do.

Pros and Cons of Perfectionism

Anaisa realised that there were far more disadvantages to maintaining her perfectionism than costs or risks associated with experimenting with changing things a bit. She realised that she feared making bad decisions or 'letting herself go' but that these were abstract fears rather than outcomes that were definitely going to happen.

	Stay as I am – not change anything	Change
Benefits	Clean and organised house	More freedom to go out and do things Less stress and anxiety More opportunities to enjoy my time with my baby Easier to accept help from others
Costs – what's the impact on my life?	I'm tired and stressed all the time My partner and I are barely speaking	I might make bad decisions if I don't think them through and these might affect my baby

	Stay as I am – not change anything	Change
	I haven't had anyone over to the house which makes me feel rude I've turned down invitations from others and they might stop asking me I'm preoccupied when I'm with my baby and I'm not enjoying myself as I'm trying to tidy up at the same time as playing I'm not doing any of the other things that are important to me – my interest in music and my swimming	I might 'let myself go' if I don't pay attention to my appearance

Over to you: try drawing out the costs and benefits for you:

	Stay as I am – not change anything	Change
Benefits		
Costs – what's the impact on my life?		

What Keeps Perfectionism Going?

Comparing Your Performance Against Others

When Anaisa did go out, she constantly compared herself and her baby to others, looking at details of other parent's appearance to see if she looked smarter than they did, comparing what people had brought with them for the baby to play with, and whether her baby was responding and moving as well as the other babies.

All babies are different and develop at different rates and in different ways. Trying to 'measure up' to other parents and babies is only going to feed a problem of anxiety, as there are infinite different ways to compare, so it is impossible to get the certainty you want – that you and your baby are doing 'perfectly'.

Getting Reassurance

Asking other people for reassurance starts off as a very reasonable and sometimes helpful thing to do – it feels nice to hear from others that they think you made the right decision, or that you are doing a good job. However, asking for repeated reassurance will increase your doubt about decisions or judgement, decrease your confidence, and increase your anxiety. See Chapter 3 for working on this.

Avoidance and Procrastination

One of the most painful downsides of perfectionism is avoiding and procrastinating – thinking that if you can't do something perfectly, then you need to put it off, or avoid it altogether.

Anaisa needed to sort out childcare for her baby for when she returned to work. She undertook extensive research online, looking at the relative merits of all the different childcare options available. She put all the information into a very neat spreadsheet on her computer, spending many hours on making sure everything was in alphabetical order, and colour coding the different options. She found it very difficult to come to a decision, and spent hours weighing up the pros and cons, feeling very anxious and thinking about how the wrong choice could affect her baby for the rest of her life. After several months of indecision, she stopped looking at the spreadsheet, and tried not to think about it, despite the deadline of her return to work looming ever closer. She avoided the decision as she could not reach the perfect answer.

Over to you: have you noticed anything that you avoid, or situations where you procrastinate or put off a decision because of a fear of not 'getting it right'?

OVER TO YOU

What Has Been the Impact of Your Procrastination or Avoidance?

What perfectionist ideas are affecting your ability to actually do this task or activity?

What could you do to break down the task you are avoiding? E.g. if you are avoiding sorting through your maternity clothes as they need to go to the 'perfect' new home (which friend, which charity shop, which recycling facility, how much to price them for online), then could you take two to three items and give them away or sell them without sorting through all of them first or coming up with the optimal plan?

And / or what ideas could you test out? E.g. if you are putting off exercise as you don't have time to do it 'properly', could you experiment with doing 15 minutes, without even putting on your gym kit?

Moving Forward: Testing Out Your Ideas About Perfectionism

Survey of Others

Anaisa believed that everyone would exhaustively weigh up the pros and cons of childcare options. She predicted that her friends, all of whom she thought were decent parents, would have multiple reasons for their choice. When out together, she asked her friends how they decided on the childcare choice for their babies.

She found a range of answers:

I went for the one which was closest – less hassle getting there.
I could only really afford the one run by my work so that was the best choice for us.

> I knew my son would really like the music group at this nursery.
> I need different arrangements on different days so went for a childminder who also looks after other children – means she'll have a bit of company too.
> My daughter is struggling with her milestones so I'm getting a nanny for the first few months, then will try a day a week at nursery to see if she can manage it.

Anaisa realised that other people were making relatively quick decisions based on practical or pragmatic reasons, without exhaustively weighing up the pros and cons. She tried to picture her baby in the different childcare options that she had visited, and thought of how much her daughter had enjoyed a big sandpit at a nearby nursery. She called to see if they had a place – she felt anxious doing this, and found herself doubting her decision, but stuck with it, and deleted her spreadsheet.

Spotting Unhelpful Thinking and Self-criticism

We have seen with Anaisa that 'all or nothing thinking' can be part of how perfectionism works. You can also look out for other 'thinking traps' when you feel anxious:

Thinking trap	Example	How it maintains the problem
Comparing	Other people find this motherhood thing so easy and I'm not so I must be a loser	Focusing on information that confirms your negative belief about yourself
Seeking total certainty	I must be absolutely sure that I am following the optimal weaning programme	Feeling pressured and self-critical – making you try even harder to get to this impossible 100% certainty
All or nothing thinking	If I can't get this all perfectly right all the time, I am a terrible mother and my child is doomed	Discounts ambiguous or somewhat positive information

Thinking trap	Example	How it maintains the problem
Selective attention	To criticism To other mothers' behaviour To baby behaviour	Reinforces your negative ideas Filters out other information about 'how the world really works'
Discounting the positive	That trip out went well but that was only luck	Reinforces your thinking that you must try harder

And watch out for avoiding things:

Thinking trap	Example	How it maintains the problem
Avoidance of people Avoiding decisions	Avoiding going out with others as a bad night's sleep means you look rough and your baby might not be calm the whole time	Prevents you finding out what would happen if you did not avoid (e.g. that people will not reject you if your baby cries) Lowers confidence

OVER TO YOU
Spotting My Thinking Patterns

When you notice these kinds of thoughts coming into your head, note them down if you can. Ask yourself a few questions to help yourself to get some distance from these critical, harsh thoughts:

Are my thoughts kind, helpful or fair?
Would I advise other parents to think like this?
When my baby is a parent, would I want them to have these ideas?

Should the Government put up public health posters saying 'Mothers: you are not doing well enough, you must get things right 100% of the time' – if not, why not? Would that be more or less helpful than a poster saying 'Mothers: you are wonderful and we cherish you' or 'Mothers: you are covered in sick and possibly poo and you are doing a great job'.

If you start to see these thoughts as just thoughts, rather than facts about your ability to be a parent, then you are starting to get away from the ideas that have kept you stuck in perfectionism.

There might be a bit (or a lot) of you still thinking that these kinds of harsh thoughts are motivating, or that punishing yourself helps you to achieve more. You might think it is 'pathetic' to be kind to yourself or offer yourself any slack. What you can do is to experiment with being less perfectionist, and less harsh on yourself, and see if you might actually prefer it. When you can think about yourself as a person with a range of values, qualities, interests and achievements, you are moving away from thinking about yourself as a performance-driven, all or nothing person, and this is likely to lower your anxiety and improve your mood. There is more information in Chapter 2 for reducing self-critical thinking.

How to Deal with Actual Criticism from Others

You may have the experience of negative comments from family members, friends or strangers. This can feel hurtful and personal and may chime with some of your self-critical thoughts. A wise person once said: 'Never take things personally, especially when they are meant personally'.

You can see that a message throughout this book is to not take things at face value. It's worth considering criticism in this way too. Useful questions to ask yourself include:

Did they intend to criticise me?

Is there any other way to interpret their remark?

Are there any other reasons they may have said what they said? Has there been a misunderstanding?

Even if they did mean to undermine me, does that say more about their weaknesses and insecurities rather than anything I've done or not done?

You may want to practise asserting yourself if this is something you find difficult. A good introduction to this and many other helpful skills can be found in the book by Dr Gillian Butler and others, *Managing your Mind*.

If someone is deliberately, systematically undermining your confidence with repeated criticism, then you may need to take action to protect yourself.

To Sum Up

- Social anxiety is very common in the perinatal period
- Self-focused attention and safety behaviours can make you feel more anxious
- How you feel is *not* how you appear to others
- Focusing outwardly, dropping safety behaviours and not judging yourself will help you to be more confident in social situations
- The idea that everything has to be perfect or right is not helpful
- You can work out and apply more helpful standards to get the best out of life and enjoy things more

7

• • • • • • •

Coping with Traumatic Experiences While Pregnant and After Birth

In this chapter you will learn:

➤ What trauma is and why it is not just *what* happened but *what it felt like to you personally* that matters most

➤ How trauma memories are stored in particular ways and can be easily triggered

➤ Why reactions to trauma often increase during this time

➤ Why your reactions to your experience make sense

➤ How to recognise if you are suffering from post-traumatic stress disorder (PTSD)

➤ How to help yourself feel better – evidence-based techniques for tackling some of the common reactions to trauma and putting painful experiences behind you

➤ Practical tips for talking to loved ones and health professionals about your experiences to ensure you are offered the right support

➤ Where to seek additional help and what kind of treatments are most effective

Introduction

This chapter will primarily focus on maternity- and birth-related traumas and how these events can impact your well-being in the postnatal period and/or subsequent pregnancies. These events are very common and include all types and stages of miscarriage as well as experiences of birth and labour. Unsurprisingly, higher rates of obstetric complications are related to higher rates of post-traumatic stress. Although never easy to go through, how you process these events does not necessarily relate to how complicated things were or how much intervention there was at the time. Even a birth or procedure seen as 'routine' or 'straightforward' by a clinician (or friends and family) may be experienced very differently by the woman herself, especially if she felt unsupported, helpless or out of control at key moments. It can feel tremendously invalidating to be holding this experience whilst the focus for others may be on how you seem physically ok now, the new baby, or a new pregnancy and how happy you 'should' be feeling.

It can feel like there is a pressure to cope and carry on with the demanding tasks of parenting, yet it takes immense energy to keep functioning and look after a new baby after trauma. For some women, even the person you looked forward to meeting most – the new baby –can be a constant reminder of the experience. It can also shake your confidence in your abilities as a new parent – often women feel their experience is far removed from what they were led to believe in antenatal classes.

After these experiences, many women struggle with feelings of inadequacy, failure and shame – unsurprising when many of the messages around us suggest pregnancy, birth and parenthood should be straightforward and completely joyful. Whilst that may mean you have struggled to talk or seek support up until now, we want you to know that you are not alone and there are ways to feel better which we hope to help you with here.

KEY IDEA

It is not what *happened but* what it meant to you personally *that matters most.*

Looking After Yourself Whilst You Work Through This Chapter

If you are coping with the effects of a traumatic experience, it is likely you are experiencing a range of reactions, some of which may feel very overwhelming, especially if you then add in the demands of pregnancy or caring for a new baby. In this chapter, we will explain why these reactions are *normal* and *understandable* as well as what you can do to help yourself feel better and come to terms with what has happened. To help explain this, there will be some examples of other women's experiences.

Very often thinking or reading about trauma can remind you of your own experience. It may trigger strong emotions or some of the other difficulties you are already struggling with, e.g. intrusive memories, flashbacks or physical sensations such as feeling sick or your heart pounding. It can feel like the intensity or 'temperature' has suddenly been turned up on your thoughts and feelings. This is especially true if you have been working hard to avoid such experiences (a very common way of coping after trauma). The sudden triggering of strong emotions and memories is a normal reaction after trauma – it is not dangerous, even though it may make you *feel* unsafe – your brain and body are simply responding to the trauma memory.

It is also normal to feel apprehensive about focusing on what has happened – you may worry you will be overly upset or won't cope. As we will explain, gradually reducing avoidance of triggers related to your trauma, and allowing your feelings and memories to surface, is an important part of overcoming your experience – with time their intensity will die down. However, it is important you go at a pace that feels manageable for you and preferably with the support of someone who knows you well. If the 'temperature' is too hot it can obviously feel overwhelming and hard to tolerate. It can also make it difficult to concentrate, stay in the 'now' and deal with the tasks in hand.

With this in mind, we would like you to take a moment to think about some ways of looking after yourself as you work your way through the chapter, in case you need them – things that might help bring the 'temperature' down a little or improve the moment for you. We will prompt you regularly to check in with yourself and how you are feeling. We would also encourage you to work through this chapter in small chunks – go at a pace you feel comfortable with – even a few minutes a day. Share it with someone you trust, if possible, so they can offer support.

In this chapter, you will be introduced to Iris and Pavarti, who have both lived through a traumatic experience that is affecting a current pregnancy (Iris) and life after birth (Pavarti). Here are some examples of their ways of looking after themselves and 'improving the moment' when they felt overwhelmed whilst working on the effects of their trauma: these are called 'grounding techniques', which help you reorientate yourself to the here and now.

I will try to ...

- Call Olivia or WhatsApp Chris
- Go for a walk or get physically active
- Smell my favourite smell
- Listen to the radio or put on some favourite music from my phone
- Remind myself that I am safe – this is my brain and body reacting to a trauma memory
- Remind myself that this is a memory; it is painful but it is in the past and is not happening again now
- Remind myself it is okay not to feel okay – my reactions are normal; they are common after trauma and understandable
- Remind myself these feelings will pass
- Remind myself that anxiety means I am human, not that there is imminent danger ahead
- Move my attention out of my head to something external to me, e.g. a picture on the wall, my baby, the rhythm of my breathing, the texture of my clothes, the sensation of being held by the chair I am in – I will gently refocus my attention on something external if it bounces back into my head.

KEY IDEA

Working on the effects of your trauma can be emotional and tiring. Going at a pace that suits you, with support from someone you trust, and thinking ahead of ways you can look after yourself, should help you to manage your emotions more easily.

OVER TO YOU
Setting up Support Techniques to Work Through Emotions and Memories Related to Trauma

What things help when you feel very upset?

Which particular people do you find supportive or helpful to speak to, be around or imagine in your mind's eye?

Are there ways you can remind yourself that your experiences are normal and understandable (like a note on your phone)?

How can you remind yourself that right now you and your baby are okay?

What simple activities might improve the moment?

Think of particular sensations which help you to feel calmer, e.g. a certain smell, the touch of something meaningful, looking at a particular picture or photograph, imagining a special place or listening to certain sounds or music.

Are there ways of refocusing your attention that help? E.g. onto your breath, onto sounds you can hear or colours you can see.

Yes but … I'm Pregnant – Is It Safe to Think About My Trauma Now?

This is not an uncommon concern for women, their loved ones and health professionals too. A recent rigorous review of the evidence for trauma-focused treatment in pregnancy found no proof of any adverse effects. The review concluded that the benefits of trauma-focused treatments in pregnancy outweigh the costs of living with high levels of stress during the remainder of pregnancy. There is also no research evidence to suggest that working on anxiety and trauma in pregnancy can cause complications.

If you are pregnant, you can decide what feels manageable for you depending on what else you are dealing with at the moment, and how much support you have from others.

What Do We Mean by Trauma?

When we talk about 'trauma', most of us will likely think of extremely frightening and horrifying situations such as an assault, a severe accident, terrorist attack, war, sexual or physical abuse. These are events that can leave a person feeling intensely afraid, helpless and / or out of control, which are all completely normal ways of feeling when something of this magnitude happens. What makes any experience 'traumatic' is how it felt and what it meant to the person going through the experience at the time. Traumatic events are often hard to talk about and think about, which makes them difficult to move past and come to terms with. It means they can have a lasting effect on your emotional and physical health long after the event has passed. Most people experience some symptoms of traumatic stress after going through very difficult events, which improve over time, but for some they do not resolve on their own. However, the good news is that the effects of trauma can be tackled, and in this chapter, we are going to show you how.

Over recent years, research has helped us to gain a better understanding of trauma and acknowledge that it encompasses a much wider range of experiences than previously thought. It can include events that are physically and / or psychologically harmful (either that you experience directly or that you witness or hear about) as well as more complex social traumas such as racism, poverty, inequality, marginalisation and other forms of prejudice and discrimination. It might involve a single event, prolonged stress or multiple events compounded over time, and can be experienced individually or collectively. Reactions to trauma also vary widely, meaning that the same event can affect two people very differently, depending on their individual characteristics and other experiences in life. Research also suggests that trauma which is caused by humans (e.g. terrorist attacks) or relational (i.e. trauma at the hands of others – often within a relationship that is needed or depended on) can be more difficult to deal with than trauma following an accident or natural disaster.

Trauma in the Context of Pregnancy and After Birth

Up until the 1990s, the trauma women experienced in the context of their maternity journey was sadly largely ignored. However, we now know many women struggle with their mental health in pregnancy, birth or postnatally, either because of past trauma or because some part of their current experience has been traumatic.

For some women there might be aspects of pregnancy or birth that trigger painful memories, leading to a re-experiencing of past trauma. Examples include a feeling of losing control over their body or of vulnerability, the need for physical examinations, or bodily pain. For others, extremely difficult experiences during pregnancy itself, such as a pregnancy loss, receiving bad news at a routine antenatal appointment, experiencing severe pre-eclampsia or pregnancy sickness (hyperemesis gravidarum (HG)) or a pre-term birth may be traumatic.

Frightening or distressing experiences during labour and birth are, sadly, a common experience which can leave women (and their birth partners) feeling traumatised long after the experience itself. This might include experiencing complications or needing intervention during birth; feeling frightened as you believed that you or your baby were going to die or come to serious harm; feeling out of control or helpless, or that those around you were coercive or didn't support you in the way that you needed. Even a birth seen as 'routine' or 'straightforward' by a clinician (or friends and family) may be experienced very differently by the woman herself, especially if she felt unsupported, helpless or out of control at key moments.

Twenty-five per cent of women will describe their birth as traumatic, and 1 in 25 of these women (around 4% of all women) will go on to develop post-traumatic stress disorder. A recent study of 650 women also found that for those who had suffered a reproductive trauma such as a miscarriage or ectopic pregnancy, 29% met the criteria for PTSD one month after the event and 18% after nine months [1].

Research also highlights that a past traumatic experience (particularly sexual trauma) can raise the risk for birth to be experienced as traumatic. In this context, common obstetric interventions, such as vaginal examinations, can trigger memories of past experiences and so trauma compounds trauma.

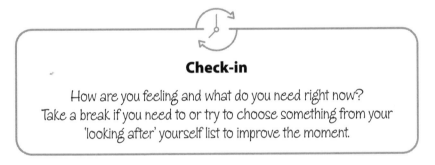

Check-in

How are you feeling and what do you need right now?
Take a break if you need to or try to choose something from your
'looking after' yourself list to improve the moment.

Coping with the Effects of Trauma During Pregnancy and Soon After Birth: Iris and Pavarti

In this chapter, we will focus mainly on examples of the experience of birth trauma; the descriptions and techniques also apply to other trauma experiences.

Pregnancy after Trauma

Iris

Iris was 22 weeks pregnant with her second baby. Her first baby was born three years ago, very early at 30 weeks, by emergency C-section, and spent 10 weeks in neonatal intensive care. His birth was very traumatic – Iris felt she was initially ignored when she noticed painful cramping in her stomach. Once she was admitted to hospital, she felt terrified. Her husband was away with work, so she was on her own. The pain of labour was overwhelming but there was a long delay before she was given any option of pain relief.

At the time, she felt self-conscious and embarrassed about the amount of noise she was making due to her pain. Several times she felt as if she was outside of her body, floating above herself, and was terrified this meant she was either going mad or dying. When her baby was finally born, he didn't cry and she thought he had died. Lots of people rushed around and in and out of the room. She couldn't see him and didn't understand what was happening. A doctor explained they had to take him for help with his breathing, before rushing out the door.

Iris felt helpless and numb. Iris and her baby eventually recovered well physically but the shock of her experience stayed with her. Although the initial flashbacks and panic attacks she was suffering with did eventually resolve, she felt she had never fully come to terms with her experience. She was a far more nervous and pessimistic person now and it had taken her and her husband a long time before they felt able to face another pregnancy.

Since falling pregnant again, Iris had noticed a significant surge in her anxiety. She had begun to re-experience intrusive memories and nightmares of her first birth experience. They often seemed to come out of the blue. Vivid images of her son when he was born would flash through her mind as well as a picture of her looking down on herself in agony and alone.

She felt tense and on edge much of the time and was having difficulty sleeping. Sometimes she noticed feeling spaced out and disconnected from the people around her. She was terrified history would repeat itself – that this baby would be born early and that he or she would die. If she felt the baby move, she would feel panicky, hot and sick. His movements often felt painful, and she would worry about what this might mean. She became increasingly overprotective of her older son and felt the need to be vigilant at all times. He suddenly seemed very vulnerable again and she berated herself for being careless if he hurt himself in the playground.

Part of Iris worried that his pre-term birth was her fault – that she hadn't taken good enough care of herself in her pregnancy and consequently she had let her son down. As far as possible she avoided talking about the pregnancy as she didn't want to 'tempt fate'. She became meticulous about keeping healthy and fit and repeatedly checked what she ate and drank for anything potentially risky to her baby. She struggled to be open with her midwives and obstetrician about her anxiety, as she didn't trust them to listen or take her seriously. She was angry about how she was ignored before and also felt let down by her husband that he had not been there for her when she was so terrified. She had little confidence that she would be looked after well this time round.

Trauma after Birth

Pavarti

Parvarti gave birth to her baby daughter 12 weeks ago. The birth was extremely fast and frightening. She noticed her initial contractions whilst she was at home with her husband and to begin with, she felt quite calm and excited. She was 10 days overdue, so was pleased that things had finally started and she was looking forward to meeting her baby.

Over the course of the next couple of hours, the intensity and frequency of the contractions increased considerably. Pavarti felt overwhelmed by the pain, scared and out of control. Her husband called the maternity assessment unit but the midwives advised Pavarti to stay at home as the contractions weren't frequent enough yet for her to be admitted to hospital. She felt helpless and increasingly desperate for more support. As she sat on the toilet in the bath-room her waters broke and pain surged. She felt terrified that something was very wrong and called out for her husband in panic. He called the midwives back who then called an ambulance.

When the paramedics arrived, Pavarti initially felt calmer but self-conscious and rather humiliated as she wasn't wearing any clothes. They examined her and told her that she was fully dilated and could see her baby's head. Pavarti again felt terrified. She had planned a hospital birth and was afraid she might tear badly or haemorrhage (as her own mum had done) without the support of midwives. Her baby was born a short time later and they were both transferred by ambulance to hospital to be checked over. Once at hospital, Pavarti felt calmer, but shocked and numb at what had happened.

Over the course of the next few weeks, Pavarti did not feel herself. She felt overwhelmed with the tasks of looking after her baby and was frequently tearful. She struggled to connect with her baby and felt guilty about this. If she sat on the toilet, she would feel dizzy, sick and in pain, which made her worry she was unwell, despite reassurance from her doctor. Pictures of her husband's shocked face when she screamed for him would flash through her mind. Any little noise or her baby crying would make her jump and her heart pound. Friends expressed envy at her fast birth. Pavarti felt unable to talk to them about how she was really feeling, as it seemed unlikely they would understand. Her husband seemed to love being a dad so she felt unable to confide in him either, as she didn't want to spoil his experience. She struggled to make sense of how she was feeling – she had had a 'straightforward' birth and healthy baby, so why did she feel so awful?

Check-in

How are you feeling and what do you need right now?
Take a break if you need to or try to choose something from your 'looking after' yourself list to improve the moment.

Common Reactions after Trauma

A traumatic experience can leave you feeling intensely afraid, helpless or vulnerable. It can shake your sense of safety about the world, your trust in yourself and others. After trauma, it is very normal to experience a range of emotions, bodily sensations and thoughts about your experience. Sometimes these experiences may happen immediately, for others (as in Iris's case) they might be delayed and only triggered (or re-triggered) later on, sometimes months or years afterwards. Sometimes you may not realise you have been affected by trauma until you are pregnant. How trauma affects you will vary from person to person, but some common experiences are described in this chapter. It is important to remember that all of these experiences are *normal reactions to very difficult events*. They do not mean you are going mad, losing control or bad in any way. Often with time these reactions will fade and what has happened will feel less vivid and less upsetting. When they do persist, there are ways of working on coming to terms with your trauma so that you can move forward, reclaim your life and feel more like yourself again.

Re-experiencing

When you have survived something traumatic, it is not uncommon to 're-experience' parts of what happened over and over again. Thoughts and images of the experience might flash through your mind or play out like a movie. These can feel very vivid, as if you are 're-living' your experience with all the pictures, sounds, smells and sensations from the time. These experiences are sometimes referred to as 'flashbacks' and can feel very unsettling and upsetting, as they often link to the worst moments of what happened to you.

At other times you might replay your experience (or some related feelings from it) in the form of nightmares, or you might find yourself suddenly experiencing a strong emotion or bodily sensation (e.g. pain) that you had at the time, without any other obvious recollection of what happened; Pavarti experienced something like this when she used the toilet. All of these experiences occur automatically and out of our conscious control. This means they can feel very intrusive and pop up even when we don't want them to or have been working hard to avoid them. Usually, these re-experiencing symptoms are triggered by something that reminds us of what has happened. These reminders could be obvious, e.g. seeing or holding your baby, returning to the hospital where you gave birth, being asked about your birth, or they might be more subtle and harder to spot, e.g. being in a particular body position, a tone of voice, a certain smell, shift in light or temperature. The connection may not be obvious to you at all, leading some people to worry that they have somehow lost their mind due to the trauma. This is of course not the case, and in this chapter we explain why you re-experience the trauma in this way and what you can do to resolve it.

Dissociation

Dissociation, or 'zoning out', in some way is a common experience both *during* and *after* a traumatic experience. Your brain decides to 'switch off', to avoid getting overwhelmed with a very stressful experience, or memories of the experience. Whilst it can feel frightening and disorientating, it is definitely not a sign of going mad or losing it, and you can learn to control it. Dissociation can range from feeling like you are on 'automatic pilot' or 'going through the motions' to completely blanking out, mental and physical collapse, or out-of-body experiences where you see yourself and what is happening to you as if from the outside looking in. Iris experienced this type of dissociation during her birth, and found it being triggered again now she was pregnant.

Dissociation (i.e. a way of mentally 'zoning out') may have been a way of coping with painful experiences in the past, and becomes more likely during birth if aspects of this experience are reminiscent of what has gone before. Dissociation during childbirth is a known risk factor for postnatal PTSD [2].

Physical Arousal

A very common experience after trauma is to feel agitated, tense or on edge, like you have to be constantly 'on guard' or 'on duty'. You may notice feeling overly alert or jumpy and easily startled. You may tremble, feel restless or have a lot of nervous energy. This can make it hard to relax and just be with your baby. Like Iris, you may feel you have to be vigilant for any sign of danger, and find yourself over-anxiously protective of your baby. Even if your pregnancy or baby is keeping you awake, you may also find it hard to sleep even when you have the opportunity. It may be difficult to fall asleep, you may wake frequently or have nightmares and anxious dreams. One of the tricky aspects of this specific reaction to trauma is that it can mirror normal aspects of your early parenting experience, e.g. feeling very vigilant to the needs and well-being of your new baby is a common experience amongst women even without any previous experience of trauma.

Difficulty Concentrating

It is not uncommon to find it difficult to concentrate, pay attention to or remember things, even if they seem simple. This can be particularly frustrating and upsetting if you are trying your best to take care of your new baby or keep up with your usual responsibilities whilst pregnant.

Strong Emotions: Anxiety, Loss, Shame, Guilt and Anger

A range of emotions are common after trauma. The most obvious is fear or anxiety – after all, this is a natural reaction to what we feel has been a dangerous or threatening situation. Your experience might have left you feeling unsafe, that life is now full of risks, that others can't be trusted or danger is everywhere – disaster could strike at any moment. Of course, trauma experienced (or re-experienced) during the course of becoming a parent means you won't just feel a heightened sense of threat for yourself but for your baby too, which will amplify your anxiety.

Another common emotion after trauma is sadness, or feeling down or depressed. Like Pavarti, some people might also notice feelings of hopelessness, tearfulness or simply feeling numb. You may have lost things that were important to you due to the trauma – for example a positive experience of pregnancy, birth or meeting your baby in the way you had hoped for. You may have lost your baby or experienced changes to your body that are hard to come to terms with. A significant issue for many women is a loss of friendships or changes in relationships if other people struggle to understand your experience, or perhaps it now feels too difficult to do the activities you hoped to do whilst pregnant or with your baby. Or you may simply find yourself feeling too low in energy or uninterested in the things you usually enjoy to get going with them again. All of this can leave you feeling that life is permanently changed for the worse, and future plans may feel unimportant or no longer meaningful to you. For example, you may have hoped for another baby or a large family, but your experiences make that feel impossible now.

Support in a Crisis

At its worst, life may not feel worth living and you may find yourself having thoughts of hurting yourself or suicide. If this is the case, please try to talk to someone you trust to offer you help and support. Support is also available through your doctor, or 24 hours a day, 7 days a week at your local A & E department or via 999. The Samaritans are also available by dialling 116 123 (free to dial and will not appear on your phone bill) or you can call PANDAS (postnatal depression and support) free on 0808 1961 776 (11 am to 10 pm, 7 days a week).

A traumatic experience can also lead to feelings of guilt and shame. You may worry about something you did or didn't do during your experience. For example, as Iris did, you may think somehow your difficult birth was your fault, that you have let your baby down, or you worry about what your actions say about you as a mother. You may think others are judging you for not achieving a 'gold standard', 'natural' birth or for how you acted at the time of your experience. Or like Pavarti, you may feel guilty and ashamed for how you are feeling now – that you aren't able to 'just get on' with enjoying your baby or bond with them. Unfortunately, unhelpful messages and opinions from those around you might leave you feeling worse or your experience invalidated, e.g. 'at least you have a healthy baby'; 'your birth was textbook!'; 'just try to forget about that and enjoy your baby'. Remember that it's *your* experience of what happened that is really key to traumatic reactions. You are the expert on you and your baby.

Irritability and anger can also feature frequently after trauma. You might notice feeling snappy or losing your temper with those close to you over simple things – unsurprising if you are feeling tired, jumpy or on edge much of the time. But you may also feel angry. You may have been hurt or mistreated. You may feel let down or betrayed by people you expected to look after you, or by those who you feel raised your expectations of a straightforward, empowering birth. If you have had a traumatic birth, perhaps, like Iris, you feel angry with health professionals for the way they treated you, with your partner for not fighting your corner or supporting you more, your friends for having a positive experience, or with your baby because they remind you of such an awful situation. Your feelings may be easily stirred up by reminders of what happened or you may feel frustrated and angry with the problems you are experiencing now as a consequence of the trauma, and find yourself dwelling on the unfairness of your experience. Anger might also be a new experience for you – it can feel confusing or frightening, especially if you have the urge to do things out of character, such as shout, swear or hit something. All of these things are understandable but can make it hard to put your experience behind you.

Shattered Confidence in Yourself, Others and the World

Before a trauma, you may have had a generally positive view of yourself, of your capabilities to manage stress and make good judgements, and of your place in the world. Trauma and your experiences afterwards can shatter these assumptions and leave you feeling completely changed. You might berate yourself for making certain choices about birth, for not coping with what has happened or for allowing yourself to think things would be okay. You might be left feeling that your 'bad' birth means that you are a bad and inadequate mother or that the world is more dangerous for you. Alternatively, you might have already had low self confidence in yourself or others and trauma during pregnancy or birth just seems to prove ideas such as 'others can't be trusted', 'bad things always happen to me', 'I always knew I would be a terrible mother', 'I'm weak and inferior compared to other people'. New trauma might open up the wounds of other difficult experiences from the past because certain aspects of these experiences overlap, e.g. being in pain, feeling in danger or vulnerable in some way. It might even feel hard to think of anything positive that has happened to you, feel that you deserve love and support or will ever be able to be happy or enjoy life again. The good news is that you can rebuild your confidence and we will help you to think about how.

Feeling Cut Off from Other People (Including Your Baby)

Many of the experiences outlined above can naturally make it hard to be in the here and now, enjoy the present or feel close to your baby and the people you care about the most. If you are troubled by flashbacks, insomnia, and have difficulties concentrating, you might be left feeling cut off or distant from those around you. If memories of what happened to you are triggered, you may experience numbness, dissociation or a sense of unreality that then gets in the way of feeling in tune with others.

Bonding with a new baby can be particularly difficult after a traumatic birth, because it can be hard to separate your feelings for your baby from your terrifying experience. You may want to withdraw from your baby because they are too painful a reminder of what has happened, or you may have been separated from your baby for a time after birth which has added to your trauma and difficulties connecting with them. They may feel quite alien to you, not like your baby – as if you are babysitting someone else's child. You may have times where you feel sure they are rejecting you or you feel angry or hostile towards them because of what has happened. You may be pregnant after a previous traumatic loss which has left you fearful of connecting with this pregnancy in some way, or your pregnancy may be retriggering past trauma that makes it hard to separate what happened from your growing baby. During times of heightened stress, our body also releases stress hormones such as adrenaline and cortisol. This can block the release of other hormones such as oxytocin, known to support feelings of closeness and connection between a mum and her baby.

You may also have thoughts that you are no good as a mother or person and consequently withdraw from relationships with your baby and your friends and family. You may feel that others simply don't or won't understand why you are struggling. This can leave you feeling alone and isolated.

Reconnecting with others is an important part of claiming back your life after trauma, especially when you have a new baby and need good support. We will show you how you can begin to do this.

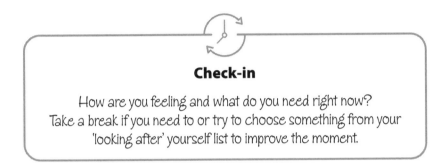

Check-in

How are you feeling and what do you need right now?
Take a break if you need to or try to choose something from your 'looking after' yourself list to improve the moment.

When Does Trauma Mean PTSD?

Post-traumatic stress disorder, or PTSD, is a specific diagnosis given when you experience certain symptoms after a traumatic experience, including flashbacks or nightmares, avoiding reminders or triggers, feeling jumpy or irritable, or having difficulties concentrating and having persistent negative beliefs and feelings. Diagnoses are often part of the process of accessing focused help in mental health services (see seeking help section at the end of this chapter). A helpful way forward right now is to find out more about the ways that your traumatic experiences have affected you.

All of the experiences described above are normal, common reactions after trauma. They can be mild or severe, brief or long-lasting. For the majority of people these experiences will resolve naturally without any long-term consequences. Not all trauma will result in mental health difficulties, and not all mental health difficulties following trauma will equate to PTSD. Having PTSD is not a weakness. Very resilient and resourceful people can develop PTSD – these are difficult experiences that can challenge any one of us in particular circumstances.

OVER TO YOU
How Does Your Experience of Trauma Affect You?

Make a note of any of these features you may experience – not everything will apply to you:

Intrusive pictures or images which flash through my mind

Flashbacks (strong memories, sometimes with a sense of feeling it is happening again)

Nightmares (these may be like memories, or dreams with themes of anxiety, loss etc.)

Strong emotions triggered when I am reminded of what happened

Strong physical feelings when I am reminded of what happened

Situations / people / words / feelings which trigger my memories, emotions and body sensations

Struggling to concentrate

Sleep disrupted (separate or in addition to disruptions caused by pregnancy or your baby)

Feeling jumpy, tense and on edge – list in which situations

Anxious thoughts

The way my confidence has been affected

The guilty thoughts which preoccupy me are …

I feel ashamed (about) …

I feel angry (about) …

I feel disconnected and cut off from …

I try to cope with my experience by …

Check-in

How are you feeling and what do you need right now?
Take a break if you need to or try to choose something from your
'looking after' yourself list to improve the moment.

Why Your Reactions Make Sense

All of the reactions you have been experiencing to date are normal human reactions to the extreme stress of trauma. It is even harder to come to terms with a traumatic experience when sleep deprived, adjusting to being a new parent or managing the challenges of pregnancy – and it works both ways: unresolved trauma can of course make the already demanding tasks of pregnancy and parenting much harder.

In this section we will delve a little further into why these reactions make sense because of the way trauma memories are made at the time, the meanings you attach to your experiences and how your body reacts when you are in danger.

The Nature of Trauma Memories

When trauma memories pop up, they tend to feel like they are happening again in the here and now rather than linked to something in the past. Due to the nature of trauma, our brains struggle to put together the experience into a coherent story and the memory is not stored like other memories.

Day to day, our brains systematically bring together and process all the aspects of our experiences – what we saw, heard, smelt, felt – and link it up with the rest of our experiences in life to form a memory that can be 'filed away' and time-stamped, so we have a clear sense of it being in the past. We might think of this like components on a factory conveyor belt being brought together and neatly packaged up with clear labels on the box of what is inside. This means the different boxes can be sorted out and stored properly until they are needed.

Try bringing to mind a recent positive experience, perhaps a birthday celebration or day out. Soon after the event, the memory of your experience feels quite fresh and detailed in your mind, perhaps the happiness and excitement you felt is easily triggered by reminders around you or when you are asked about it. You may have discussed it with others or spent time thinking about it and looking at reminders. Over time, your brain moves the components of your experience around the conveyor belt, processes and packages it up so that the vividness and emotional intensity linked to the memory begin to fade. Once stored away, the experience is not forgotten but is unlikely to intrude into your awareness very often. However, it can be easily recalled in a clear way if you want to think or talk about your experience again.

When something traumatic happens, your brain is flooded with stress hormones and overwhelmed by the task of trying to respond to the threat facing you. It struggles to bring the different aspects of your experience together and process what is happening. Imagine the factory conveyor belt again. It's as if some components are too hot, too rough, too big or some might be missing altogether. Your brain is trying hard to do what it needs to do but the nature of the experience means it simply can't be brought together and neatly packaged up in the same way as the experience outlined above. Consequently, parts of your traumatic experience are stuck on the conveyor belt going round and around. They are 'raw' and unfinished, waiting to be processed. This means they can be easily triggered and intrude into our mind when we don't want to be thinking about them. They might feel full of gaps, jumbled up or like they simply don't make sense.

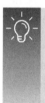

KEY IDEA

Trauma memories aren't put together like other memories. This means they can be easily triggered and you can feel like you are 're-living' your experience, which can be frightening and upsetting.

Your Thoughts and Beliefs About What Happened

Another key factor driving your experience now will be the way you made sense of what was happening to you *at the time of the trauma* **and** the *conclusions you have come to since* about yourself, others, the way the world works and perhaps your future. Identifying the thoughts which lie behind your emotions can help you make sense of how you are feeling. Often the meanings attached to an experience at the time are not accurate or helpful but will be understandable given what we believed was happening at the time, and due to the influence of our past experiences.

Let's look at Iris's and Pavarti's stories for some examples. They both had frightening thoughts and beliefs at the time of the trauma, and formed conclusions afterwards about what the trauma meant about them, others and their future.

> At the time of her trauma Iris thought she was either going mad or about to die. At one point she also feared her baby had died.

When these very intense and terrifying thoughts occur in the middle of a trauma they can be 'too hot' to be processed. These thoughts can keep coming back in the intense way they were felt at the time, even though you know that they are not true.

> Since the trauma, Iris had come to the conclusion that other people (especially health professionals) couldn't be trusted, that she was a careless and irresponsible mother and that bad things were bound to happen again to her and her children (including her unborn baby).

This constant sense of being unsafe kept her in a state of threat.

> At the time of her trauma, Pavarti also feared she or her baby were going to be injured – she worried she would have a terrible tear or haemorrhage. Since the trauma, Pavarti believed she was a bad person for not bonding with her baby and for feeling so upset about her 'straightforward' birth. She believed other people were judging her and that it was going to be impossible to enjoy parenthood.

All of these ideas meant it was understandable that Pavarti and Iris were stuck with feeling afraid, angry, guilty and unsafe.

OVER TO YOU

What has your experience been? Can you spot any thoughts you had at the time of the trauma or since which might explain how you have been feeling? We will come back to this so try not to worry if this feels too difficult now.

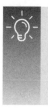 **KEY IDEA**

Strong emotions after trauma, such as anxiety, guilt and anger, are very common. The way you think about the trauma and what it means to you can help to make sense of these feelings.

How Your Body Reacts to Danger: It Holds the Score

As described earlier in the book, our bodies prepare us for action when we are in danger or afraid. This involves a host of physiological changes which drive a range of physical responses. We may notice tension in our muscles, our heart racing, feeling breathless, feeling trembly and startled as a consequence. Our brains take note of dangerous situations so that we are prepared for similar situations in the future.

After a traumatic experience, our brains can continue to behave as if there is danger, long after it has passed. Our bodies continue to react so that you are ready to fight or flee. This can leave you feeling jumpy, vigilant and on edge – it is as if you are stuck in survival mode. Another response is 'freeze', where you may feel unable to move or may dissociate (zone out). These are protective mechanisms designed to keep us safe and avoid us getting overwhelmed.

KEY IDEA

*Unpleasant physical feelings make sense because your body may still be responding **as if** there is danger long after the trauma has ended.*

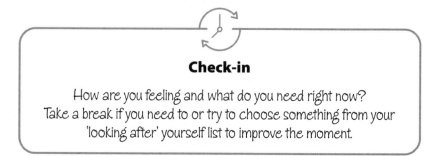

Check-in

How are you feeling and what do you need right now?
Take a break if you need to or try to choose something from your 'looking after' yourself list to improve the moment.

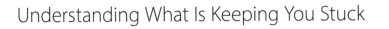

Understanding What Is Keeping You Stuck

Trying to cope with the effects of trauma as well as look after yourself in pregnancy or care for a new baby is extremely hard. Understandably, you will adopt different strategies to try and manage how you are feeling and get by. Whilst some of these may help you cope in the short term, in the longer term they can stand in the way of feeling better.

Avoiding and Blocking Memories

It makes sense that you would want to try and avoid or control upsetting memories or thoughts if they cause pain, discomfort, unease or signal danger. Unfortunately, avoiding memories stops your brain from doing what it needs to do to get the memory in better shape. Pushing thoughts and memories away is a bit like pushing parts off the conveyor belt – the memory can never get fully put together, so gets stuck and replays over and over. If you think about it, it's not something you do with other sorts of memories, which naturally fade in intensity over time.

It is also a very tiring strategy – it takes a lot of mental effort, which can be extremely challenging if your resources are already depleted from caring for a new baby or the physical demands of pregnancy. What is more, trying to avoid memories can have the opposite effect:

> For the next sixty seconds we want you to try your absolute hardest to think of anything but pink elephants. You can think about whatever you want just NOT pink elephants.

What happened? Were you successful? Or did you have at least one (or more) occasion(s) where an image of a pink elephant popped into your mind? Most people report this. Usually, the harder we try to block out a particular thought, the more preoccupied we become. So, while this strategy is understandable, it is actually counterproductive.

Avoidance of Memory Triggers

If you are aware of specific activities that remind you of what has happened or trigger your trauma memories, you will very likely try to avoid these too.

This can be really difficult after a traumatic birth, as your baby will likely be a strong reminder of your experience, as can antenatal or postnatal appointments, perhaps because they involve returning to the site of the trauma (e.g. hospital) or because you have to interact with health professionals similar to those involved in your trauma.

To manage, perhaps you have handed care of your baby over to someone else when you can, or zone out / detach when they are around. You might choose to avoid or cancel hospital appointments or limit your interactions with health professionals. Again, these are natural ways of coping with a traumatic experience and do not say anything about you as a person other than you are trying your very best. In the short term they may alleviate some distress, but longer term they will also stop your memories of what happened being fully processed and filed away as something in the past.

Vigilance for and Avoidance of Risk: Taking Extra Precautions

After trauma, it is natural to experience a heightened sense of danger because your experience has made you more aware of risk and how things can go wrong. You may find yourself scanning or repeatedly checking for danger, feeling extra vigilant, 'on guard' or taking extra time and effort to analyse the risks of a particular situation in a way you wouldn't have before the trauma. You may also avoid situations you feel are risky for fear of history repeating itself or disaster striking again. Or you might take extra precautions to keep you and your baby safe.

Being on high alert or avoiding situations you fear are risky might seem sensible – it is natural to want to protect yourself and your baby. However, it is likely that the avoidance and extra precautions are making it hard for you to live the life you want. When you act 'as if' you are in danger, you continue to feel in danger. So these strategies often have the opposite effect of what you hope they will achieve – they feed your sense of threat and stop you from recognising evidence you are safe. See Chapter 3 on unwanted intrusive thoughts for more on safety-seeking behaviours and how to tackle them. This is a very common issue after trauma.

Dwelling on What Has Happened: Rumination

After something traumatic has happened, it is natural to go over what took place in your mind as you attempt to make sense of your experience. This can be helpful if it brings a new, less threatening perspective. However, many people find themselves dwelling on thoughts and questions about what happened for long periods of time. Thoughts and questions like 'Why … ?', 'What if … ?', 'If only … ', 'I should … '. You might think over what you or others could have done differently to prevent the trauma, or how you could have reacted differently. For other people their thoughts may focus on what they have lost and how things have changed. When these kinds of thoughts pop up and send you around in circles in your mind, it is likely you are dwelling on what has happened in an unhelpful way – we call this type of thinking 'rumination'. It often feels quite automatic and can be hard to stop. Dealing with it is important though as it can leave you feeling bad and might maintain unhelpful ideas like 'I will never get over this'. It may also stop your memory from being fully processed, as it effectively keeps the conveyor belt going round and round but with nothing being processed.

KEY IDEA

Some of the ways you try to cope with your memories, thoughts and feelings may keep you stuck and stop you from coming to terms with what has happened – identifying this will help you work out what you can do differently to support you moving forward.

OVER TO YOU
What Strategies Can You Spot which Might Be Keeping You Stuck?

Are you using any of the following to try and feel safe or come to terms with what has happened?

Avoiding situations, people or places	
Avoiding or suppressing thoughts or memories	
Dwelling on what happened with lots of 'What if', and 'If only' thoughts	
Scanning for certain dangers or danger more generally	
Repeatedly checking, e.g. your baby, the lock on your front door	
Seeking reassurance	
Any other precautions you have spotted?	

Check-in

How are you feeling and what do you need right now? Take a break if you need to or try to choose something from your 'looking after' yourself list to improve the moment.

Moving Forward: How to Feel Better and Start Coming to Terms with What Has Happened

There are three main areas we focus on when helping someone overcome the effects of their trauma:

1. Getting the trauma memory in better shape so it can be fully processed and filed away
2. Addressing the meanings which have been attached to what happened to you that drive strong emotions such as fear, guilt, anger and shame
3. Tackling avoidance and other strategies such as rumination, which keep the memory and meanings stuck

Reclaiming Your Life: What Are You Working Towards?

Before we take you through some of the focused techniques known to help alleviate the impact of trauma, we want to encourage you to think about what is important to you and what you would like to be doing more (or less) of, or what you would like to start again, even if it is not possible to do it in exactly the same way as before.

This is important, because after a trauma, people often feel that life has changed or they have been robbed of what matters to them. Starting to try to claim these things back is an important part of overcoming the effects of what has happened, rebuilding your life and feeling more like yourself again.

This can be hard if you had hopes and expectations about how your pregnancy or time as a parent with your new baby might be, and it feels like the trauma has affected this. Alongside the trauma, the challenges of early parenthood or pregnancy can also feel hugely stressful or overwhelming – even the simplest tasks may feel impossible at times.

Let's look to Iris for an example:

> Before becoming a parent, Iris described herself as a relaxed and easy-going person. She enjoyed going to the gym and socialising with her friends. She cooked with her husband or they went out for dinner together occasionally. After the trauma of her first birth and navigating the transition to first-time motherhood, Iris felt like a completely different person, lost and confused amid a sea of new demands and emotions.

To help her start to think about reclaiming her life, Iris asked herself the following questions:

How did I used to spend my time?
What did I used to enjoy?
What made me feel good?

What would I like to do now?

What have I stopped doing that I would like to do again?

What could I do instead of the things which are impossible now?

Iris began to make a list of the things she valued and would like to work towards doing more (or less) of or start again. She also included some new activities she was keen to try out once her baby arrived.

Here are some examples from Iris's list:

Free Time / Hobbies

Listen to some of my favourite albums

Find a new box set to watch that I might enjoy

Work / Study

To finish work on time and not work at home

Home Life

Have dinner out with Pete or cook together at home at least once a month

Allow Pete to cook for me

Arrange a babysitter so we can have some time together alone

Parenting

Plan some activities just me and Harry

Dedicate some time to play at the weekends

Order what I need for the new baby

Research baby groups I might like to try when the baby arrives

Relationships

Contact Clare, Jana and Catherine for a coffee or catch-up

Health / Exercise

Reduce my excessive checking of food and drink

Some of these felt like big goals but she thought about what was possible to start now; which first active steps she could take towards these goals today. She was careful to think of specific things which felt manageable to her:

1. I will send Clare a message to see if she is free for a coffee
2. I will Google a local restaurant for Pete and me
3. I will text Jana about borrowing her 'next-to-me' crib

She would revisit her 'reclaiming my life' goals each week to check in with her progress and set herself some new tasks for the week ahead.

OVER TO YOU
Reset Your Goals

Spend some time thinking about the same questions as Iris. Write down your thoughts about the things you would like to do more of, less of or start again.

What would help you to feel more like yourself again?

Now think about what you could do right now to start to work towards claiming your life back. Take one step at a time. Start simple and choose some small specific actions that feel manageable to you today.

For example, if you would like to do a group with your baby, you might start by Googling what options are available or joining a local Facebook group to ask other mums.

My goal is	First steps towards this are

Tell a loved one or friend what you intend to do if you think that also might help motivate you and try to check-in with your goals regularly, thinking about the next steps you can take.

KEY IDEA

Looking for opportunities for small but meaningful steps to reclaim your life after trauma is an important first step to feeling better.

Getting Your Trauma Memory in Better Shape

Allowing Your Memories to Come and Go

The memories of any traumatic experience are always horrible and upsetting. You will probably want to avoid, suppress or turn away from them as much as possible. At other times you may naturally get caught up in all the 'whys ...?' and 'what ifs ...' of what happened. As we saw above, these are common and understandable reactions but have a downside – they stop your brain doing what it needs to do to fully process and file the memory away.

But what's the alternative? Let's look at Pavarti's experience as an example.

Pavarti was experiencing intrusive memories of her traumatic birth in a number of ways – often pictures of her husband's shocked face would pop into her mind and at other times she would suddenly re-experience the same physical feelings she had at the time of her labour, e.g. dizziness and sickness, particularly if she was sitting down or on the toilet.

Pavarti tried her best to suppress these thoughts and feelings. She would shake her head and try and think of something positive, but usually the pictures and feelings just popped straight back up again. She noticed the more she was trying not to think and feel these things, the more her mind just bounced straight back to the memory. She accepted it might be helpful to try out a different approach. After all, she was working really hard to try and get rid of the memories but her efforts weren't paying off.

Pavarti experimented with doing less when the memories appeared. Instead of working hard to suppress them she did her best to just let them be. To notice that they had popped up but to try and wait for them to pass. She found it helped to imagine them a bit like unwanted guests at a party – annoying and definitely unwelcome, but usually less disruptive if she just noticed them and let them be rather than trying to wrestle them out of the door. It wasn't always easy and certainly took practice but Pavarti gradually began to find it easier to stand back and do less when the thoughts popped up. She noticed that the memories seemed to be coming a bit less frequently and certainly passed more quickly this way.

Another simple strategy Pavarti found helpful was to label the memories as memories when they appeared and to remind herself that these were events from the past. She told herself that when they do pop up, it is an opportunity for her to help her brain do what it needs to do rather than something dangerous to try and avoid.

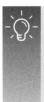

KEY IDEA

Doing less to your memories when they pop up, i.e. letting them come and go, will help them be processed and stored away like other memories.

Check-in

How are you feeling and what do you need right now? Take a break if you need to or try to choose something from your 'looking after' yourself list to improve the moment.

OVER TO YOU
Working on Unwanted Memories

Are there memories or flashbacks that you notice yourself working hard to suppress or avoid? Or perhaps you get tangled up in arguments with yourself about the 'Whys?' and 'What ifs'?

Could you experiment with a different approach? Is it worth finding out what happens?

Over the next few days try to treat your memories a bit differently – perhaps you can label them as Pavarti did, 'just memories' or 'unwelcome guests'. Or you might find another metaphor helpful to think about – visualising intrusive thoughts and memories as:

- 'Clouds passing over in the sky'
- 'Leaves floating by on a stream'
- 'Trains passing through a station'

The key point is to do whatever helps you to stand back and observe them rather than trying to push them away, control them or get caught up in analysing them.

Remember this isn't a quick and easy task. It can take some practice and it is very natural to find yourself back in old well-rehearsed habits, trying to suppress or churning the memories over. So be gentle with yourself and try again when you are able. Like breaking any habit, consistency and repeated effort will help.

Tackling Memory Triggers

Step 1: Finding the Triggers

The nature of trauma memories (i.e. that they are still 'raw' and 'unprocessed' and untethered in your thinking) means they are usually easily triggered. They pop up frequently, often when you don't want to be thinking about what happened, and bring strong emotions from your past trauma into the present.

As we saw earlier, that might be as an image or flashback, body sensation, smell, taste or simply a strong emotion without any other obvious recollection of what happened. It can feel really disorientating and worrying. They can make you feel unsafe, even when you are otherwise feeling okay, or you might feel sudden waves of shame, humiliation or some other feeling when there is no apparent reason to. Sometimes this might come 'out of the blue', but at other times there may be an obvious situation or experience which has reminded you of what happened, e.g. a birthday or anniversary of a particular occasion, visiting the hospital where you gave birth, an antenatal scan, interacting with your baby, seeing someone involved in the trauma (including your partner), talking about what happened or seeing / hearing / reading about something similar on TV, the radio, in a book, magazine or via a podcast etc.

Understanding what triggers the memory for you is an important step towards making sense and gaining control over your reactions, as well as putting the memory in the past. Some triggers will be subtle; others are more obvious. Usually, they are simple everyday things which remind you or in some way 'match' your experience during the trauma, e.g. a similar smell, colour, voice tone or facial expression. This can trigger a memory without the connection being obvious, as the threat system operates by there being a similarity rather than a perfect match with what happened during the trauma. This matching process is over-inclusive, which is one reason why some people have lots of flashbacks.

Once you have a good idea of what triggers are an issue for you, the challenge is to help your brain put the threat in the past and be able to take in the present as safe. We will show you how to do this. Let's look again at Pavarti's experience as an example.

> Pavarti experienced a number of unwanted memories of her birth. She would often see a vivid image of her husband's shocked face as he came into the bathroom when she shouted out for him. She also experienced bodily sensa-

tions that she had at the time – sometimes she felt sick, dizzy, and a dragging pain in her stomach, and at other times she felt a sense of panic and her heart pounding. All of these were extremely vivid and often left her feeling like she was either back at the time of her birth re-living her experience or in danger. The picture of her husband's face would generally come into her mind out of the blue, even if she was feeling quite calm and relaxed. The physical sensations felt more obviously triggered by sitting in a particular position or hearing a particular sound, e.g. her baby or another baby cry, or sirens blaring.

As a first step, Pavarti kept a diary of the times parts of her memory were triggered over the course of a week. She kept an audio note on her phone of (1) what was triggered; (2) where she was and (3) any similarities she could spot between this current situation and the trauma.

Some triggers were quite obvious to her and often made her apprehensive. For example, sitting on the toilet. Others were more subtle, e.g.:

Her husband's facial expression when they were watching a film together
Her body's position as she bent over to put on her shoes whilst sat on a dining
    chair
The time of day
The colours green and yellow (similar to the paramedic's uniform)
The smell of the bathroom air freshener

She found it particularly helpful to spot the more subtle triggers – she now had a better understanding of why she could feel ambushed by strong feelings or flashbacks without any warning.

Here is an extract of her diary:

Day	What was triggered?	Where was I?	Similarities between this and my trauma
Monday evening	Vivid image of Shashi's shocked face	Watching movie	Time of day, alone with Shashi, his facial expression

Day	What was triggered?	Where was I?	Similarities between this and my trauma
Tuesday morning	Feelings of dizziness, sickness, pain in my tummy	In the bathroom using the toilet	Sitting on the toilet, in the bathroom, no underwear
Wednesday afternoon	Flashback to lying on our bed. Paramedic examining me	Playing with Aisha in the living room	Colour of baby clothes matches paramedic's uniform
Thursday afternoon	Several different flashbacks – seeing myself in the bathroom, the bedroom etc.	Having a coffee with Paula, talking about how I was feeling about Aisha's birth	Talking directly about things that happened

KEY IDEA

Spotting memory triggers can help you make sense of and begin to gain control of your reactions.

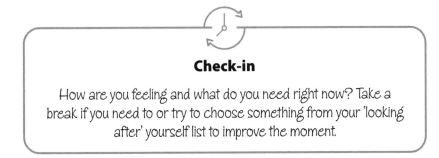

Check-in

How are you feeling and what do you need right now? Take a break if you need to or try to choose something from your 'looking after' yourself list to improve the moment.

OVER TO YOU
Noticing Your Memory Triggers

First off, are there any obvious memory triggers which spring to your mind like they did for Pavarti? Make a list if you can and use the checklist below to help you.

- Places where the trauma happened or those similar to it?
- Talking about what happened or having to write something about it?
- Anniversaries or particular dates?
- People involved in the trauma or people who look similar to those with you at the time? For example, health professionals, your partner, your baby
- Certain sounds?
- Certain smells?
- Certain lights or colours?
- Facial expressions?
- Tones of voice?
- Being touched in a particular way or place on your body?
- Reading about or hearing about similar experiences, e.g. on TV, the radio, a podcast or in the newspaper?

Next, try to see any memories popping up from now on as an opportunity to work out what sparked them. We know this isn't always easy. Take your time and just do what you can.

If a memory is triggered, remember to remind yourself this is just the trauma memory, and it is in the past. You are safe and not in danger now.

Try to keep a note over a few days to see what you can notice, just as Pavarti did. Do this in whatever way is easiest (jot it down, write a note on your phone, record an audio message to yourself, or tell your partner or friend so they can keep a note for you).

Remember the three questions to ask yourself are:

1. What has been triggered?
2. What was the situation? (Try to be as detailed as possible to help you answer question 3)
3. What similarities between then and now can I spot?

What have you learnt from this exercise?
Did anything surprise you or help you make sense of how you have been feeling?

Step 2: Breaking the Link between Then and Now

Armed with more information about her triggers, Pavarti set about trying to break the link between the memory trigger (i.e. what was similar *now* to her past experience) and her trauma (what happened *then*). Up until now, she had worked hard to avoid the obvious triggers where she could, and often felt she simply automatically looked away or took herself out of the situation. Whilst this had helped a little in the moment, she still often felt overwhelmed by memories of her birth. She realised now there were many more subtle triggers she hadn't spotted, and avoiding all of them would be impossible. She decided to experiment with a new strategy – she knew it would take some courage but she reminded herself of how much she was struggling now and how she wanted her life to be different.

She set about gradually mentally approaching the triggers and deliberately focusing her attention on all the *differences* between then and now. She looked for differences in what she could see, hear, smell, touch as well as who she was with, what she could do and the time of day etc. She started with one of the weakest triggers (e.g. her baby's yellow clothing) before moving on to the more challenging ones (e.g. being asked about her birth). With time, practice and support, Pavarti found she was able to work through a number of triggers, and she noticed herself automatically shifting the focus of her attention to differences if a memory was triggered unexpectedly.

Memory Trigger: Baby Clothes (The Colour Yellow)

Then	Now
Paramedic wearing yellow	*Aisha* wearing yellow
Night time	*Day* time
Smell of disinfectant	Smell of my *hand cream*
In the bedroom	In the *lounge*
I am lying down	I am *sitting* down
I am in pain	I feel *no pain*

Then	Now
I am in labour	I have *given birth and am safe*
Several people	I am *alone* with Aisha
No radio	*Radio on*
No baby toys	*Baby toys* all around me
Unable to move	I can *stand up and move around*

Memory Trigger: Talking About My Birth Experience

Then	Now
I am in my traumatic experience	I am talking about my *past* experience
Several people, no Paula	I am *with Paula*
Night time	*Day* time
I am outside	We are *outside*
I feel hot	I feel *cool*
Lips dry	*Lips wet* with coffee
I am lying down	I am *sitting* down
I am in pain	I feel *no pain*
I am in labour	I have *given birth and am safe*
Quiet	Chatter and coffee shop *sounds*
No Aisha	*Aisha* is here in the buggy
Unable to move	I can *stand up and move around*

KEY IDEA

You can gain control over your reactions and speed up processing of the trauma memory by focusing in on all the differences between then and now when the memory is triggered.

Check-in

How are you feeling and what do you need right now? Take a break if you need to or try to choose something from your 'looking after' yourself list to improve the moment.

OVER TO YOU

Then versus Now

Have a look back at your list of memory triggers. Start by rating them from weakest to strongest. You can use any scale you want – whatever makes sense to you, e.g. 0–10, 0–100 etc.

Choose one of the weaker triggers as a starting point to practise 'then versus now'. It is easier to spot differences if you aren't pulled all the way into the memory.

What might you need to help you practise approaching this memory trigger?

- Do you need someone to do it with you?
- Or perhaps something specific to practise with, e.g. a particular sound to play or a smell to recreate.
- Do you need to create more differences to help you? E.g. put some music on, open a door or a window, stand up rather than sit down (or vice versa).
- Or perhaps having something to ground you in the now might help (see the section 'Dealing with dissociation – grounding' for more information on this).

Remember the task is to do your best to stay in the present and really zoom in on all the differences you can see and to practise this as often as you can. If it helps, write down some of the common differences you tend to spot somewhere accessible (e.g. a card you carry in your wallet or your phone) to help focus you in the moment. The more you can practise this technique repeatedly and consistently the more quickly you will move your memory into the past, feel more in control and have less things remind you of what happened.

Dealing with Dissociation: 'Grounding'

Step 1: Tracking Dissociation

Iris experienced dissociation during and after her trauma. During her birth she had an 'out of body' experience where she felt like she was floating above herself. Afterwards she also noticed having episodes of feeling spaced out or disconnected from the people around her, including her young son. She found these quite unsettling and worried about her state of mind. Her husband often expressed frustration at the times Iris seemed to 'zone out' and not be listening to him or responding to their son.

Iris and her husband learned that the episodes Iris was experiencing were dissociation and were normal after trauma – she was not losing her mind or being rude. Her brain had learnt to dissociate during her birth and was now using that same strategy again as a way of coping with heightened stress and reminders of what happened. To help Iris better understand the triggers for her dissociation and the first signs that she might dissociate, she kept a note of the triggers she spotted and the first signs of her dissociation experience.

Iris spotted that common triggers for her dissociation were her son crying (or hearing another baby cry), feeling under pressure (e.g. when she was in a stressful work meeting), hearing a scream on the TV or radio, anticipating an antenatal appointment or feeling a painful movement from her baby. The first sign of an episode tended to be her vision feeling blurry and out of focus and sounds around her starting to seem distorted or further away.

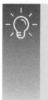 **KEY IDEA**

Dissociation is a normal reaction after trauma but can feel disorientating and frightening. You can start to tackle it by looking for the first signs of dissociation and potential triggers.

Check-in

How are you feeling and what do you need right now? Take a break if you need to or try to choose something from your 'looking after' yourself list to improve the moment.

OVER TO YOU

Spotting Triggers for Dissociation

If you experience episodes of dissociation like Iris, try to spot what happens at the time (or just before) you dissociate. Note a few typical examples down if you can, to help you. This is the first step to gaining better control of dissociation.

Here are some questions to help you begin to think about your examples and spot the triggers:

> Who were you with?
> What were you doing?
> Were you very busy or doing very little?
> How were you feeling?
> Under pressure or stressed?
> What were you thinking about?
> Was there an obvious reminder of your trauma present?
> What were the first signs of dissociation?
> Was there a feeling in your body?
> Did things around you look or sound different in some way?

Step 2: Gaining Control of Dissociation

To help her gain control of these episodes, Iris adopted some grounding strategies designed to reorientate her to the present and remind her she was safe. These included wearing and squeezing a locket her husband had given her since the birth of her son; focusing hard on something around her in the here and now – sometimes something she could see, e.g. a picture on the wall, sometimes something she could feel, e.g. the arms of a chair or texture of her clothes, sometimes something she could hear, e.g. the traffic outside or birds in the garden. Moving to stretch her body also seemed to help when she could.

OVER TO YOU
Bringing Yourself Back from Dissociation

Once you have a better idea of dissociation triggers and the first signs of 'trouble', we want you to have a think about anything which might help you connect with the here and now – i.e. things that 'ground' you and pull you out of the memory.

This might be shifting the focus of your attention, as Iris did, to something you can see, touch, smell or hear; using an object, image, smell or body position / movement. Anything that helps you to feel safe and connected with the now. Often a meaningful object, soothing smell or image that you have acquired *after* the trauma is most helpful – something you associate with being safe, calm and helps remind you the trauma has passed, and life has continued in a way you feared it might not at the time.

Choosing a strategy that maps the nature of a trigger can also be helpful, e.g. if you notice a smell triggers dissociation, try out a grounding smell; similarly, if a body position, sound or certain touch triggers the experience for you, try to find an alternative that you associate with safety and feeling soothed.

It is usually helpful to experiment with different strategies and try these out one at a time when you are not dissociating, so that you can feel more confident they are easily accessible to you when you need them. You might choose to use different strategies for different situations (e.g. being at home versus in public) and you might also want to consider recruiting someone to help you, e.g. a partner or friend. If they spot the signs of dissociation, you might have an agreement of what they will do to help you re-orientate yourself to the now, e.g. they might squeeze your arm, say your name, remind you that you are safe etc.

Here are some examples of other people's grounding strategies to help you think about what you might like to try for you:

Attention

Press my feet firmly into the floor and remind myself I am safe
where I am
Name one thing I can see, hear, smell and touch
Rub the fabric of my top back and forth between my fingers
Squeeze my special key ring

Smell

Smell the lavender oil I bought with mum
Smell my husband's new aftershave
Smell my new perfume
Rub the hand cream Hannah gave me for my birthday over my hands and
inhale deeply

Images

Bring to mind the sea, the sounds and smells of the waves and sand, the
warmth of the sun
Imagine Toby's birthday party – his happy grown-up face looking healthy
and strong

Phrases

We are safe
This is a normal reaction to an abnormal event
I am strong and capable
People believe in me

Objects

Squeeze my new car keys
Rub the ring mum gave me

Movement

Stretch myself tall and big

Hug my knees in and rest my head

Rotate my ankles and feet

Move like I couldn't at the time – stand up, dance around

Make a fist and squeeze repeatedly (particularly helpful if you suffer a faint
response; see the chapter on blood-injury phobia for further work on
overcoming fainting)

KEY IDEA

*Grounding strategies can help pull you out of the memory and
into the present.*

Check-in

How are you feeling and what do you need right now? Take a
break if you need to or try to choose something from your 'looking
after' yourself list to improve the moment.

Tackling Nightmares and Night-time Memory Triggers

If you find trauma memories are keeping you awake, remind yourself
you and your baby are safe and the trauma is over. Use your grounding
strategies (see 'Over to You: Bringing Yourself Back from Dissociation') to
bring your attention back to the now. It might be helpful to try and spot the
memory triggers and focus on all the differences with now.

If you are woken up by a nightmare or bad dream, remind yourself they
are coming from the trauma memory. You are safe and not in danger.

Again, use any grounding strategies that might be helpful and support from a partner or loved one if that is helpful. Try to run the images from the dream on and give them a new ending which fits with what you know now, i.e. that the trauma is over, and what you are able to do now. If you are experiencing a recurrent nightmare or bad dream, it can be helpful to think about a new less frightening ending in the day time and to practise rehearsing it in your mind's eye at a time when you feel less anxious.

Recounting Your Experiences: Talking Through What Happened

The Benefits

After trauma, talking or thinking about what happened can feel daunting and painful. You would probably prefer not to talk or think about it, but as we described above, actively avoiding talking about it can prevent your brain processing the experience in the required way for the memory to be 'filed away'. It is also stressful and effortful to have to keep concealing or suppressing what happened to you, and may not be proving very effective at reducing your distress.

There are many potential benefits to going through your experiences. Research shows that expressive writing about emotional experiences can be beneficial for your health, including reducing pain, improving sleep and increasing performance in the workplace. Telling your story of the trauma should help your memory become more organised, which in turn can help you to make better sense of what happened, e.g. by joining up the parts that, perhaps until now, felt jumbled up; noticing the parts which feel most upsetting to you and why; filling the gaps with new information you might have remembered or gathered from other sources; and giving your experience a beginning, middle and end so it is 'time stamped' as happening at a particular time and place rather than just a series of worst moments that keep coming back to haunt you.

In telling your story, you might also recognise your own personal qualities and strengths within your experience or feel a sense of accomplishment in being able to face what happened with such courage.

You might find that it is possible to find new meaning in what happened or recognise that what you feared at the time did not come to pass. New information might help you to take a different perspective on yourself, others or the worst moments of your experience that then helps to alleviate some of the pain you feel. Again, it can help to 'time stamp' these aspects of the memory ('this is what I thought *then* but this is what I know *now*') and consequently it will feel more like it is in the past. You could choose to express what you know now or these new perspectives in a way that make them stand out from what happened then, e.g. writing them in a different colour, font or texture etc.

Here is an example of Iris's updated account of her trauma:

> '… in labour I was screaming and had the thought that people are judging me and think I'm weak and crazy. I know now that it is fine to make as much noise in labour as you want! Some friends have told me that they screamed the house down at points …. At the moment my baby was born I was in such pain I thought I was going to die … I know now that I got through this moment and it did not last forever … I thought the baby was dead … I know now I have a healthy happy baby who I care for well, I was dissociating then, which is not going mad, it's your body protecting you from an intense situation … everyone was rushing around but speaking to each other not me and I felt lonely and uncared for … I know now they could have done a better job of communicating and it was not my fault, but they were focused on the medical situation as my baby was in distress …

Telling your story can also help you to connect with external support and in doing so normalise and validate your reactions and shift feelings of self-criticism and shame.

How to Go Through Your Experiences in a Manageable Way

In CBT, telling your story will be done in quite a specific and detailed way and we call this 'reliving'. It is difficult to attempt this without the support of a therapist.

Here we are talking about creating a narrative of your experience that enables you to express what happened. The key idea is to try and turn towards rather than away from the memory so you can begin to process it and be able to acknowledge and recount your experiences when you choose to, without being overwhelmed.

Telling your story can take many forms – you might write about it, talk about it or create some other representation of it, e.g. a piece of art, creative writing, music, dance or poetry. There is no right or wrong and you can experiment with different methods to work out what feels best for you.

When you are describing your experiences, it is helpful to tell the facts of what happened but also try to express the thoughts, feelings and other sensations you had at the time. You might also consider how your experience connects with how you think and feel about yourself and others now and other past experiences too.

Other people might support you by listening and encouraging you in this process but also by filling in gaps if they witnessed something you were not able to (e.g. your partner, a midwife or medic) or helping you to make sense of certain experiences that felt confusing or frightening at the time. Your midwife should be able to advise you on how you can arrange a meeting to go through your birth experience and have any questions you might have answered where possible. Finding out as much as you can about what happened can help you piece your story together and bring in new perspectives. For example, you might gather new information that contradicts what you feared was happening at the time.

Of course, you may not choose to share your account with anyone else yet but if you do, think about who is best to hear it with the compassion and empathy it deserves. Someone you trust to keep you safe and not blame or shame you. Sometimes this might be a partner or family member but there are many reasons why that might not be possible, and you may want to ask a friend. Try to choose someone you trust to listen, be supportive and offer a helpful perspective.

You will need to recount your experiences at a pace that feels manageable for you. It is probably helpful to work on it a little at a time rather than all in one go. You want to try and choose a time if you can when you feel you won't be interrupted or distracted, you feel in a safe place and where possible can be supported by someone you trust (either in person or remotely). Think about the resources and skills you have built up already that might support you to stay in the present rather than being pulled into the memory (e.g. through a flashback or dissociation). You might want to spend some time really focusing in on the differences between then and now before you begin, and have any grounding objects within easy reach. When you begin to pull your story together, start with what you can remember. If there are gaps, it might be possible to make sense of these once all the bits you do recall are together in one place or with the help of other people. Try to end your account at a point you felt safe.

Remember it is likely to feel upsetting and painful to some degree – that is natural, but by allowing yourself time and space to think about what happened, those feelings should become less intense over time.

Finally, try not to compare your experiences with other people's. Remember it is not the extent of the trauma but the impact it has had on you which matters most – having compassion for what happened to you and how it has affected you is really important. Try to also remember this story is only a part of you. It is awful that it has happened but there are many experiences before and after it which continue to make up who you are.

Tackling a Heightened Sense of Danger

When something bad or dangerous happens or nearly happens, it is natural to feel more at risk. You may also feel your baby is more at risk, or perhaps this has generalised to other loved ones too. Whilst most of us can accept that risk is a part of life and that bad things can happen, usually we don't dwell on this or think it is particularly likely it will happen to us. We get on with life with relative ease. However, trauma shines a spotlight on risk and can make us believe that things that previously felt unlikely are now bound to happen to us – things feel more dangerous than before.

You may have developed new beliefs following your experiences:

'No one can be trusted to protect me or my baby'

' Danger is potentially everywhere'

'I need to be on guard or disaster will strike again'

'I'm weak and vulnerable; I can't cope'

You may also notice your behaviour changing to try and help you feel safer from the dangers that you now believe are present or more likely. You may begin to avoid certain situations or you might take extra precautions where previously you didn't feel it was necessary, such as checking things repeatedly or seeking a lot of reassurance (if repeated checking is a problem for you, you may also find the ideas in Chapter 3 on unwanted intrusive thoughts helpful). We call these behaviours *'safety-seeking behaviours'* because they are natural ways of seeking safety when we feel in danger. However, the downside is that if you do them when the danger has passed, they usually keep feelings of threat very high because (a) they keep you focused on risk and (b) prevent you from finding out if your fears are true. It would be like a solider returning from a war zone who continued to carry a gun and wear combat gear.

As we have also seen, when memories of the trauma are triggered, this can also bring the feelings of threat you had at the time of your experience into the present. So, a heightened sense of danger is stirred up by your memories, your thoughts and your ways of coping with feeling unsafe. It can take time for this feeling to settle down and it usually will. However, if you find yourself seeing danger everywhere, trying overly hard to keep yourself, your baby or others safe, exhausted from feeling constantly on guard and consequently not being able to get on with life and motherhood in the way you wanted, then the ideas in this section may be helpful to you.

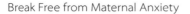
Let's look at Iris's experience as an example.

> Iris's traumatic first birth had left her feeling very unsafe in this pregnancy. She felt tense and on edge all the time and grew very protective of her unborn baby and young son. She was constantly vigilant for risk, e.g. in her body, or in the playground, and trying very hard to keep everyone safe. It felt like her body's 'alarm system' went off constantly.

Why is this understandable?

Firstly, Iris was experiencing frequent intrusive memories and nightmares of what happened to her and her first baby, which naturally brought with them the feelings of threat and terror she had experienced at the time.

Secondly, Iris had a number of thoughts of danger which preoccupied her – for example *'it is naïve to think pregnancy and birth can be straightforward'; 'history is bound to repeat itself'; 'professionals can't be trusted to care for me properly'; 'I need to do everything I can to stay safe or I will lose this baby'; 'danger is everywhere, I'm careless and need to stay alert'*. With these thoughts on her mind, she was bound to feel anxious and at risk.

Thirdly, Iris was working exceptionally hard to stay safe – she was taking lots of precautions (such as being very meticulous with her diet and over exercising), avoiding certain situations (such as talking to her midwife or obstetrician) and scanning for danger wherever she went. These strategies meant she was exhausted, constantly on edge and not able to find out if certain fears were true (e.g. that her current care team wouldn't listen). At other times she found that she was so focused on one particular danger (e.g. whether her son's car seat was belted properly) that she would nearly miss others (e.g. a red traffic light). Naturally this left her feeling shaken and more anxious, as it just added evidence to the idea that she needed to stay alert and be extremely careful.

So, we can summarise what keeps feelings of danger going after a trauma a bit like this:

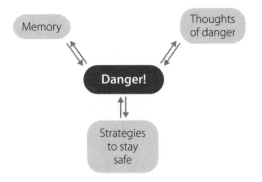

KEY IDEA

A heightened sense of danger is fed by trauma memories popping up, thoughts of danger and your ways of coping.

Over to You: Working Out What Is Keeping Your Sense of Danger Going

Have a look at the questions below to help you map out what factors are contributing to your heightened sense of danger.

1. What situations, places or people tend to make you feel unsafe now?
2. When parts of the memory pop up, do you find yourself feeling unsafe or in danger? What memory triggers have you spotted so far?
3. When you feel that something is unsafe or dangerous, what sorts of thoughts are in your mind?
   - Do you feel more vulnerable or less able to keep you and / or your baby safe in some way?
   - Have you lost trust in your judgement or your ability to cope if things go wrong?
   - Does your baby seem more vulnerable to you now?
   - Have you lost trust in other people, do they seem less reliable or able to keep you safe? Or do they frighten you in other ways?

- Does the world seem generally more dangerous?
- Does it feel that it is better to treat most things as risky than be sorry?
- Does the future seem blighted by danger?
- Does it feel like you are now bound to attract bad things, that being happy will tempt fate or that worse things are likely to happen to you?

4. Are there ways you are coping with feeling unsafe which might unintentionally be contributing to how anxious you feel?

- Are you scanning for danger or hypervigilant in some way?
- Are you on the lookout for certain things?
- Are you repeatedly checking your baby is okay? How does this leave you feeling?
- Are you avoiding certain situations? Altogether or in part? How does this cause difficulties for you?
- Do you tend to look out for evidence that something bad is likely to happen? Or go over worst-case scenarios in your mind? How does all this leave you feeling?

Make a note of your reflections and have a go at filling in your own summary below:

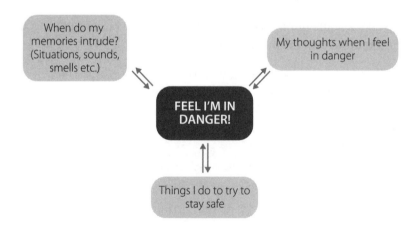

Now we have an idea of what is contributing to your heightened sense of danger, let's focus on what can help dial it down. Back to Iris.

Iris had already learnt about memory triggers. She understood how certain things in the present which resembled her trauma in some way could set off flashbacks, physical feelings in her body or periods of zoning out. She had learnt to spot the triggers and was practising 'then versus now' and 'grounding' techniques to help break the link between the memory of her past trauma and what was happening currently. Whilst this had helped and her intrusive memories were less frequent, she still noticed that she was often scanning for danger, avoiding situations and preoccupied with feeling unsafe.

To begin to tackle her thoughts of danger and less helpful ways of coping, Iris tried out a number of different things. A lot were about experimenting with doing things differently – dropping her safety-seeking behaviours, reducing avoidance and scanning for danger to help her test out her anxious predictions. Others included keeping a log of all the times she expected the worst but things turned out okay and gathering good-quality, reliable information about the likelihood of another pre-term birth and other risks to her and her baby in this pregnancy.

Let's look at some examples of what Iris tried out.

Moving Forward: Testing Things Out (Anxious Predictions, Reducing Avoidance and Dropping Precautions)

In CBT, we use the term 'behavioural experiments' to describe what we do to test out, in a planned way, our beliefs about how the world works. When you are feeling anxious, the beliefs you are putting to the test are usually in the form of a prediction about what will happen when you act against your anxiety and do something differently, e.g. don't avoid or use a standard safety-seeking behaviour. Remember beliefs are theories, not facts. They are usually understandable conclusions that you have come to because of your experiences, but may be holding you back now if you apply them very rigidly.

The idea is that these experiments will help you to find out that the things you feel most anxious about do not happen in the way you fear, highlight how safety-seeking behaviours can be counterproductive and enable you to discover how the world really works and hopefully move on with your life.

Iris – Experiment 1: Testing the Idea 'Professionals Can't Be Trusted to Care for Us Properly'

Iris believed with near certainty that health professionals couldn't be trusted. This meant she was avoiding talking openly at her antenatal appointments and was constantly on the lookout for examples of women not being listened to or health professionals getting things wrong. However, there was also a part of her that recognised that this meant she was always on edge at appointments and not getting the support she needed in pregnancy. Here is the experiment she planned to help her begin to evaluate her current professional network more fairly.

Before the experiment, Iris wrote down what she planned to do and specific predictions about what she believed would happen. She rated how likely, right now, she felt they were to happen.

What am I going to do?	What am I testing out?
At my next antenatal appointment, I will mention my anxiety when I am asked how I am	*My anxiety will be ignored – it will not be acknowledged (90%)*
	The midwife won't make eye contact with me (80%)
	She will only focus on how the baby is (95%)

After the experiment Iris reviewed her predictions and wrote down what actually happened. She reflected on what she had learnt and what this meant for her moving forward.

What happened?	Were the predictions true?	What did I find out?
The midwife asked me how I was. She paused and looked up at me and gave me time to talk, and she listened. She asked me about what help I was getting and what I felt I needed	No	This midwife seems concerned about me. Not all health professionals behave in the same way. I feel a little lighter for sharing. Some support is available. I could try to be more open again

Iris – Experiment 2: Testing Out the Impact of 'Scanning for Danger'

Iris was in the habit of constantly scanning / checking for danger to try and feel safer. She felt like she needed to be 'on guard' 100% of the time, otherwise she might miss a risk and something bad would happen to her, her son or her unborn baby. However, she also found it very tiring to be 'on duty' like this all the time, and noticed that she was missing things anyway because of being so vigilant (e.g. in the car). She decided to experiment with what happened if she did things differently.

The following is what Iris wrote down before her experiment:

What am I going to do?	What am I testing out?
When I walk to the gym I will do my best to pause my scanning for danger and try to refocus on my walk and what I want to do in the gym On my walk back I will do what I usually do – look out for every possible danger around me	I will feel more anxious if I'm not on the lookout for danger (100%) Something bad will happen to me if I don't keep constantly checking (80%)

What happened?	Were the predictions true?	What did I find out?
Nothing bad happened I felt more anxious on my walk back from the gym I tripped up on the curb when I was concentrating on the crowd ahead of me and trying to work out how rowdy they were	*Scanning for danger makes me anxious Scanning for danger does not eliminate risk Scanning for danger makes it harder for me to concentrate and take in everything around me I need to try and check / scan less*	*No*

Iris: Keeping a Note of When Things Turned Out Okay – Challenging 'Emotional Reasoning'

One process that can keep a sense of threat going is something psychologists call *emotional reasoning*. This happens when you conclude that how you are feeling proves something is true, despite possible evidence to the contrary.

Since her trauma, Iris often had the feeling that something bad was about to happen. It kept her on the lookout for danger and often meant she checked things repeatedly, e.g. if her little boy was okay. To help her evaluate how accurate her feelings were, Iris kept a note of each time she had the 'bad feeling' and did her best not to respond to the feeling (i.e. check) so it would be a fair test. She asked herself what she was afraid would happen in that moment and then noted down how things turned out. Over the course of a week, Iris noticed the feeling every day, sometimes several times a day, but nothing bad happened on any of the occasions. She concluded that her feelings were not very accurate and probably not a helpful guide of how in danger she and / or her children really were.

Iris: Examining the Idea that 'History Will Repeat Itself'

After trauma, it can feel very likely that something terrible will happen again. This can be particularly difficult if you are pregnant again after a previous trauma. It can be useful to find out if your estimates are accurate, and even if there is a risk, whether there are things you know now that can reduce your risk or increase your confidence in your capacity to cope.

Iris was fearful that history would repeat itself. She *felt* certain she would have a second pre-term and difficult birth. Her feelings were telling her it was 100% likely. She knew from discussions with her midwife and obstetrician there was an increased risk that her baby would be born early because of her experience first time around, but they had emphasised that it was not a foregone conclusion. Iris recognised she was overestimating her risk of a second pre-term birth and this was naturally driving up her anxiety.

When she felt worried, she found it helpful to remind herself 'Whilst there is an increased risk, this is not as likely as it feels, and certainly not a given'; 'My feelings are not a reliable guide to how risky something is', and she also tried to refocus on her present. She also believed that a second pre-term birth would be as awful as before and that she wouldn't cope. To help her evaluate these ideas, Iris considered all the things she knew now that she didn't know then that might help her to make different choices and put plans in place to feel better supported. (See Chapter 8 on pregnancy-related anxiety for more on this).

Tolerating (Some) Risk and Uncertainty

After trauma, it is easy to feel plagued with doubts and feelings of uncertainty alongside thoughts of risk and danger. Many find these feelings unbearable. Consequently, your anxiety might set you the impossible task of being 100% sure of things to keep safe. Naturally, you then strive for certainty and try to eliminate all risk, only to find yourself faced with more doubts, more anxiety and greater and greater limits set on what you can and can't do. It is a horrible vicious cycle that has the potential to create many more problems than it solves.

Uncertainty and risk are a part of life that we all have to live with, and you will have managed this well in many situations (e.g. if you have ever been in a car or crossed a road). No-one can guarantee to you that no bad things will ever happen again, and of course, when it comes to having babies, there are factors which elevate risk. However, what is guaranteed is that *trying to be absolutely sure* about your or your baby's safety only leads to more anxious suffering. It rarely helps to make anything feel more certain or predictable.

Learning to tolerate some risk and sit with some uncertainty is therefore an important part of tackling your anxiety and reclaiming your old self after trauma. Accepting this can of course feel especially difficult if you are pregnant or have a young baby – naturally you want to do your absolute best to keep them safe. The system around you might also bombard you with messages of risk and your responsibilities as a parent can leave women feeling like they have all of the responsibility (and not always all the control) for keeping their baby safe, which then drives up fear and anxiety and the urge to try harder to keep safe.

As Iris did, it is important to try and find out if you might be overestimating the likelihood of something bad happening again, and consequently trying too hard to eliminate all risk or uncertainty in a way that creates more problems than it solves. Using good-quality, evidence-based information is key here. Try to avoid general searches online. It is also important to consider whether you are underestimating your ability to cope if something difficult were to happen again, as this will also add to your anxiety. Are there things you know now and support you have now (or could be put in place) which might build up your belief in your resilience? It might also be helpful to think about other areas in your life where you are able to tolerate uncertainty better, and what helps you do that (e.g. how a meeting might go at work; what the weather will be like tomorrow). Or perhaps there are people you know who do this well – think about what helps them or better still ask them. You might want to think about whether you are approaching uncertainty in an all or nothing way, e.g. if something is uncertain, then something terrible is bound to happen. What evidence do you have that doesn't fit this idea? As Iris did, it might be useful to consider evidence of when things have felt risky or uncertain but turned out okay, or if not, how you have coped better than you imagined. This doesn't mean you have to 'accept' that something bad will happen, it's just remembering that you can get through difficult situations. For more ideas on how to build up your tolerance of uncertainty, please see Chapters 2 and 3 on tackling repeated worry and unwanted intrusive thoughts.

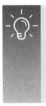

KEY IDEA

A heightened sense of danger can be tackled by experimenting with doing things differently and evaluating your thoughts of danger.

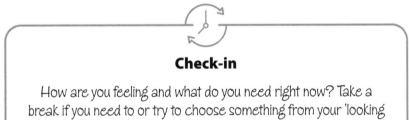

Check-in

How are you feeling and what do you need right now? Take a break if you need to or try to choose something from your 'looking after' yourself list to improve the moment.

OVER TO YOU

Evaluating Thoughts of Danger and Doing Things Differently to Put Fearful Thoughts to the Test

Look back at the specific thoughts and ways of coping you identified that might contribute to your heightened sense of danger. Would it help to try and treat these ideas as theories rather than hard facts? To check out how reliable your feelings are as a guide for what will happen? To see what happens if you reduce avoidance or other precautions or try to dial down hypervigilance or scanning for danger?

- What do you need to do to evaluate how accurate these ideas are and how helpful your methods of coping are?
- What evidence would you need to see?
- What evidence do you already have that doesn't fit your fears?
- Are you relying too much on your feelings as evidence for how risky something is? How could you find out?
- Are you overestimating the likelihood that something bad will happen? Who could help you understand the actual risk?

Setting Up Your Own Behavioural Experiments

Behavioural experiments are the best way to put ideas and theories to the test. Remember the idea is not to put you and / or your baby in real danger. The focus is on being able to do the usual things you would have done had you not experienced the trauma. Here are some tips for making them as helpful as possible:

1. Choose a situation which usually feels risky, e.g. letting my baby be held by someone else so I can do something for myself. Try to pick something in line with your reclaiming your life goals so it feels meaningful and helpful to tackle.
2. Start with something that brings on the anxiety but isn't overwhelming – i.e. an experiment you will learn from but is also realistic to complete right now.
3. What are you trying to test out – what are your anxious predictions about this situation? E.g. 'They will drop her.'
4. What do you need to do to fairly test this idea – what usual precautions do you need to drop, e.g. allow someone else to hold her (reduce avoidance); try to resist the urge to tell them what to do; go and make myself a cup of tea rather than stand and scan for signs they may be about to drop her.

5. Note what actually happened – was your prediction true?
6. Think about what you found out and what you have learnt. What does your experiment tell you about your beliefs, your ways of coping?
7. How can you take this further?

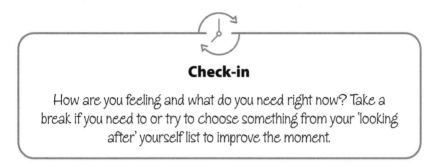

Check-in

How are you feeling and what do you need right now? Take a break if you need to or try to choose something from your 'looking after' yourself list to improve the moment.

A Note on Panic Attacks

A panic attack is a sudden rush of physical sensations in your body which build to a peak within a few minutes. These sensations might include your heart racing, pain in your chest, breathlessness, feeling lightheaded or dizzy, sick, trembly, that you are dying, going crazy or losing control. The sensations can feel very uncomfortable and frightening, but it is important to know they are not dangerous. It is your body reacting normally to fear. Panic attacks often happen after trauma, when a situation or experience reminds you of what happened. The trigger may be obvious to you or sometimes they can feel like they have come out of the blue. More information on dealing with panic attacks can be found in Chapter 5.

Further information on tackling self-criticism can found in Chapter 6.

Re-connecting with Others and Building Your Relationship with Your Baby

We saw above that it is natural to feel disconnected, isolated or alone after trauma, and yet good support is vital for feeling better and managing with a new baby. You can test this out in the ways we have described earlier, and see also the sections on connecting with your baby in Chapters 7 and 8 for lots of practical ideas on how to approach this in pregnancy or postnatally. You may want to connect with others who have had a similar experience. See the 'References and Resources' section for specialised organisations and peer support.

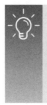

KEY IDEA

It is natural to feel disconnected from other people and your baby after trauma but there are ways you can build those connections up again.

OVER TO YOU
Connecting with Your Baby and Others after Trauma

Are there ways in which you feel less connected with the people who care about you or your unborn baby or children? What barriers have you noticed to feeling more connected?

Are there particular fears, anxious predictions or judgements of yourself getting in the way, e.g. 'People think I should just get over this and pull myself together – there's no point in talking about how I feel'; 'I can't trust others to support me'; 'If I let myself love my baby I will lose them'; 'I don't deserve any support'; 'It wasn't "love at first sight" so there must be something wrong with my ability to bond with my baby.'

Are there ways in which the memory being triggered makes it hard to be in the now or connected with your baby or someone else close to you? E.g. flashbacks, dissociation etc.

Are there other things getting in the way such as certain ways of coping? E.g. for Iris, she was so preoccupied with keeping healthy through what she ate and exercise that there was little time for others.

All of the strategies we have spoken about to date, i.e. working on memory triggers, tackling a heightened sense of danger with behavioural experiments, grounding strategies for dissociation and so on, should help to create more opportunities for connection. Have a look back at these sections if you feel it might help to revisit them.

Tackling Guilt and Shame

As we discussed earlier, common painful feelings after trauma include guilt and shame. These feelings might be triggered by reminders of what happened, or guilty and shameful thoughts you are struggling with now. Guilt is usually focused on feeling bad about something you did (or didn't do) – you feel regret and remorse; shame usually follows fearful thoughts of being intrinsically bad or immoral as a person. You may feel ashamed of some way you or your body reacted during the trauma, or how you have behaved since. You may beat yourself up for things you did or didn't do or feel, blame yourself for what happened or feel you have let people down including your baby (e.g. not giving them the start in life you wanted or having the 'perfect' birth). You may worry that others are judging you as a consequence or find comments from others confirm your guilty or shameful thoughts, e.g. 'at least you have a healthy baby'. It can feel hard to let go of guilty and shameful thoughts, but these are rarely helpful or productive in the long term.

Iris believed her difficult birth was her fault and that she had let her baby down. She believed she should have been more assertive when she was first in pain, and that if she had been, he would have had fewer difficulties breathing. She also believed she should have taken better care of herself in pregnancy. She thought she was a bad mother for not seeing or holding her son immediately after he was born, and that she should have fought harder for this. She worried this meant their relationship would always suffer. She was also concerned about what the doctors and midwives thought about her because of how much she had screamed through her contractions. She believed she deserved to be left in pain and wonders if looking back they were punishing her for being such a 'drama queen'.

Pavarti felt ashamed about how she was feeling now. She felt certain it showed she was a bad mother. She knew her birth was quick and straightforward so she kept telling herself she should be happy and 'just get on' with enjoying her daughter. She worried other mothers in her antenatal group thought she was ridiculous for being so upset and would probably reject her if she was honest about how she was feeling.

Consider:

- If Pavarti or Iris were friends of yours, what would you want to say to them?
- Would you agree with their thinking or take a different view?
- Is there another explanation for how Iris behaved and how Pavarti is now feeling?
- Are they treating themselves fairly or judging themselves too harshly?
- Are there any advantages to their guilty or shameful thinking?
- What do you imagine the downsides might be?

OVER TO YOU
Tackling Your Feelings of Guilt and Shame

- What do you feel most guilty or ashamed about?
- Can you spot any 'I should …' or 'I shouldn't…' type thinking when you look back at what happened?
- Are there ways in which you feel you 'fell short' of your standards during or after the trauma?

Consider the Impact of These Thoughts

- What impact are these thoughts and feelings having on you, your life and relationships (including with your baby)?

- If you woke up tomorrow and were able to feel less ashamed or guilty, how would life be different?
- What are the potential benefits of tackling these ideas? For you? For your baby? For your future?

Building a Fairer Perspective

Now you have an idea of what thoughts lie behind your guilt and shame and how they impact you, we want you to try and work towards an alternative view.

The questions below are designed to help you start to loosen up your thinking. As always, ask someone to help you consider these questions if it feels difficult to pull back and put in a different perspective by yourself.

1. If this was a friend's experience, would you agree with the conclusions they had come to? Why?
2. Is it possible you are taking on too much responsibility for what happened?
3. Are there other factors you are ignoring that are important to consider? If feeling very responsible for some aspect of what happened is distressing you, you may find it useful to look at Chapter 3 on unwanted intrusive thoughts for an exercise specifically aimed at tackling an inflated felt sense of responsibility.
4. Is it possible you are relying too much on your feelings as evidence, e.g. feeling ashamed therefore you must deserve to be?
5. What other evidence is there to consider?
6. Are you looking back with the benefit of hindsight – are there things you know now which you could have never known then which mean your conclusions about yourself are not fair?
7. If you had acted differently then, how much would things have really changed? Are you overestimating the likelihood it would have been a better outcome? Is there anyone you could ask to help you find out?
8. Are there any good or understandable reasons for why you acted in the way you did?

9. Were there any benefits from what you did or didn't do which you may be ignoring – again consider asking someone if you think this might be helpful.

10. Is it possible that the feelings or behaviours you feel ashamed about are normal and understandable reactions to extreme stress? How could you find out?

Taking all of the above into account, what is a fairer, more balanced and helpful way of looking at things?

When you feel guilty or ashamed, how could you remind yourself of this point of view so you stop ruminating and refocus on other things? Would it help to keep a note of your more balanced view, the key evidence for this and why it matters to let go of shame? Where would you keep this note so it is accessible?

Check-in

How are you feeling and what do you need right now? Take a break if you need to or try to choose something from your 'looking after' yourself list to improve the moment.

Tackling Anger

Anger is another very common and understandable emotion that many people experience for some time after trauma. It can also be an emotion that feels a bit frightening or daunting, especially if it is out of your usual character and / or you are looking after young children. No-one should experience trauma, so it is natural to dwell angrily on how it might have been prevented or who / what might be responsible. Your anger may be telling you that you have been mistreated, abused, wronged in some way, violated, treated unfairly or let down by those you expected to care for you – that your needs weren't fully met.

Your anger might be directed towards individuals, an organisation as a whole or sometimes it might also turn on yourself. We saw that Iris was justifiably angry with health professionals for ignoring her needs, her husband for not being with her when she needed him most and herself for some of the actions she took in pregnancy and during birth. However, over time, anger can prove costly and work against you, damaging relationships, prolonging your suffering and keeping you from moving on with your life. For Iris, anger was continuing to affect her relationship with her husband and that with her new midwife and obstetrician.

Choosing to let go of anger can feel difficult, even if you know it is causing problems for you. You may think this is 'giving in', 'weak' or letting others off the hook.

> Iris was worried that by letting go of her anger about how she had been treated during her first birth she was somehow telling herself that what happened was okay, that she doesn't care and she is a 'push-over' for not fighting harder.

Would you agree with her? Why?
Is accepting a situation has happened the same as agreeing with it?
Does Iris need her anger to prove she cares and that she is not okay with what happened? What might working on her anger say about Iris as a person?
Is she weak? Or is it a sign of strength and courage?

OVER TO YOU
Breaking Free from Anger

What Am I Angry About?

Take a moment to think about your experience of anger and where it is focused.

Here are some questions to help:

How does my anger present itself, e.g. do I hold it in, try and squash it down, do I simmer away in my own head or do I express it in some way?
What do other people see when I am angry?

How do I feel it – in my body? In my mind?
What triggers it?
What am I most angry about?
Who am I most angry with?
Why do I believe they behaved in that way?

It might be the actions of someone at the time, someone's actions since, or both. It might spill out to other people too who weren't directly involved, e.g. family and friends that you feel don't fully understand or support you in the way you need. You may feel angry with your baby for 'causing this' if your birth was difficult. You might also feel anger about the consequences of the trauma for you – things you have lost, e.g. joyful time with your baby or in pregnancy. Remember these are all understandable and common ways to feel after trauma.

Now take a moment to think about how the anger affects things for you. Ask yourself:

How Does Anger Affect Me?

What impact is anger having on me personally?
How is it affecting those around me?
Has my anger helped in some way? Has it helped other people to change their behaviour? Or not?
In what ways does my anger make life more difficult for me?
What does it stop me from doing or enjoying fully?
If my anger disappeared, how would life be different?
What concerns do you have that make it difficult to let go of your anger? Are there any ways of answering these concerns or other ways of looking at this?
What might you say to a friend or what would a friend say to you?

Ask someone for support in thinking this through if that feels helpful.

Letting Go of Anger

It may feel too effortful to commit to changing your anger right now. When you are ready, there are some tips below that might help. Remember, working on this when you are ready shows courage and strength.

First off, ask yourself (use your answers above to help you):

How would you like your anger to be different?

What are some specific benefits of committing to tackling your anger? How and who will it help?

What feel like the most important reasons for trying to tackle this now?

What are the costs of your anger now? What does it risk in the future?

The next step is to make a plan of some alternative ways of responding to and expressing your anger.

Iris began by trying to practise catching herself when she was in her head, angrily ruminating about how she was ignored and let down. She tried to respond with compassion for herself – recognising and acknowledging her anger, that what happened was not okay and it was natural for her to feel this way. But she reminded herself that continuing to hold onto her anger had costs for her and her relationships and kept her away from the life she wanted to be leading (e.g. that it kept her irritable and distracted; took up valuable energy and kept her in the past rather than focusing on the future with her family).

She did her best in these moments to redirect her attention – to get out of her head and into activities she valued, e.g. time playing with her son, exercise, calling a friend, finding a new recipe to cook and so on.

She also decided to try and find some constructive outlets for her anger – ways she could try and use her experience to help others. She joined her local Maternity Voices Partnership (MVP) so she could try and work together with other parents and providers of local care to improve services for other women (see www.nationalmaternityvoices.org.uk for details of your local MVP).

She also shared her experiences with other women via organisations such as the Birth Trauma Association (www.birthtraumaassociation.org.uk) and Make Birth Better (www.makebirthbetter.org). Finally, Iris decided to write a letter to the care team that looked after her during her first birth. Her intention was not to send it, more to express her feelings – she wrote about her anger about their actions, the impact it had had on her, how and why she had decided to move on and what she felt this said about her as a person.

What feels possible for you to do right now? What can you do as a first step? Who could support you with this? You may feel sceptical that anything will help. That is okay. The important thing is to just try out new ways of responding or expressing your anger, to see if this helps.

Coping With the Loss of Your Baby

If your loss has been complicated by trauma, then it is likely you will benefit from the support of a therapist, to help you make sense of your feelings and work out a way through them. The scope of this book does not allow us to give the in-depth attention these issues deserve, but we hope you may find some of the exercises outlined already in the chapter helpful.

If you have experienced the traumatic loss of your baby at any point during pregnancy, birth, or soon afterwards, then in addition to the experiences above, you will likely also be trying to manage intense feelings of sadness and grief. Everyone experiences grief differently – you may feel anger, numbness, intense sorrow, guilt or relief. There is no right or wrong answer and it can take a lot of time to come to terms with the shattering loss of your pregnancy or baby. It can be a slow and painful process to rebuild your sense of self and find meaning and direction in life again. There is no set timetable for this.

It can also be useful to talk about your feelings of grief with a loved one or to think about ways you might like to respect the memory of your baby whilst balancing first steps to re-engaging with your life when you are ready. Some families choose to create a special place for their baby, create a memory box or choose a particular way to mark anniversaries or birthdays that feels meaningful for them. Try to take care of yourself too – it can be easy to neglect your basic needs when you are grieving, but this is only likely to make your pain worse.

We have provided a list of organisations offering support to families after the loss of a child in the 'References and Resources' section at the back of this book, which we hope will be helpful to you.

Coping With Persisting Pain and Physical Injury After Birth Trauma

A traumatic birth can result in physical injuries which can be life changing. This might include perineal trauma (a cut or tear between the vagina and anus), nerve damage, pelvic floor damage due to overstretching or tearing, pelvic organ prolapse, spinal injury, and, on rare occasions, a brain injury. You may also have scarring or ongoing pain as a consequence of your birth. Sometimes people experience ongoing pain even if the physical damage has healed. All of these things can act as potent reminders of your experience, trigger trauma memories or frightening images of what you fear might be happening in your body. In turn, this can intensify physical discomfort and pain or draw your attention back to your body. You might also feel low in mood and dwell on the way your body has changed and the things you have lost. You might avoid activities for fear of being reminded of your injuries or exacerbating your pain, but find yourself all the more preoccupied with what has happened rather than moving forward with your life. In addition, your injuries might have left you feeling unsafe and vulnerable, meaning you put extra effort into staying safe but end up feeling overly alert and anxious.

If you have experienced a physical injury during birth and / or have ongoing pain, it is important you are offered the appropriate treatment and pain relief. Talk to your doctor, midwife or obstetrician about your options. You may wish to arrange a birth reflections meeting, to go through what happened in order to better understand what caused your injury. It might help to write down your questions in advance with the support of your partner or a loved one. You may also want to make a complaint. Birthrights can help to guide you through your options (www.birthrights.org.uk). The organisation MASIC (Mothers with Anal Sphincter Injuries in Childbirth) also offer a freephone birth injury helpline on 0808 164 0833, to listen and signpost.

Coping with the effects of a physical injury or pain after birth isn't easy. However, it is important to try not to give up on the things you value. There may be things you aren't able to do now and it is, of course, important to acknowledge this loss, but it is also important to recognise what you are able to do, what hasn't been lost and what you can begin to build back into your life. There may be activities from the 'reclaiming your life' section here which can help to prompt you over what first steps you might want to take towards something you would value doing. Building up activity gradually should also help to boost your mood, your physical strength and shift your focus away from pain and injury and unhelpful ruminations. Of course, it is important to pace yourself and get to know your limits, so experiment with new things gradually.

OVER TO YOU

Rebuilding Your Life After a Birth Injury

Consider:

- What injury or injuries have you suffered?
- What is the worst thing about the injury for you?
- Are there things you have lost because of your injury? What do you miss the most?
- What do you fear your injury says about you as a person and / or your future?
- What do you avoid because of your injury or pain?
- What precautions do you take because of your injury or pain?

Now Also Think Carefully About:

- What are you still able to do?
- What activities might you value or enjoy (either with or without your baby)?
- What manageable first steps could you take to build some of these back into your life?
- Who could support and encourage you? What would it be helpful for them to do?
- If pain is triggering trauma memories (or vice versa) could you practise then versus now?
- If you are putting extra effort into staying safe, are there any behavioural experiments you could try here to put your fears to the test? See the section 'Tackling a Heightened Sense of Danger' in this chapter for some ideas on how to do this.

Check-in

How are you feeling and what do you need right now? Take a break if you need to or try to choose something from your 'looking after' yourself list to improve the moment.

Supporting Someone Coping with the Effects of Trauma During Pregnancy or After Birth: Top Tips

You may be reading this chapter as you are concerned about your partner or someone else close to you. Keeping these points in mind may help you:

- It can be upsetting and confusing to see someone suffering after a traumatic experience.
- Try to educate yourself on the range of normal reactions after trauma – a good start is to read this chapter.
- Recognise that seeking help and talking about feelings during pregnancy or after birth can take great courage – women often fear being judged or

having their baby taken away. Give space to listen when they are ready without judgement.

- Understand that aspects of pregnancy and birth can be traumatic for women, even if they seem straightforward to you or others.
- Understand that the effects of trauma are tiring – tiring on top of the exhaustion they may already be feeling because of pregnancy, recovering from birth or caring for a new baby.
- Assure them their experiences are human, normal and understandable, and that you are there to support them.
- Gently remind them that they are safe and the trauma has passed, if they are feeling frightened or are reliving some aspect of their experience.
- Support with baby care where possible.
- Encourage them to do things that are meaningful to them, little by little.
- Help them to spot any memory triggers and focus on all the differences now.
- Ask them about any grounding strategies that might be helpful for you to support with.
- Support them to focus on evidence of their strengths, and resilience and capacity to cope.
- Remind them why you think differently to their blaming, guilty or shameful thoughts.
- If they are angry, remind yourself they are not angry with you but what has happened to them.
- If they seem distant or unloving, remind yourself this is a common reaction to trauma. Assure them you are still there for them.
- Partners can also experience post-traumatic stress after a birth, as well as other reactions. If you also feel affected by what has happened, do try to seek help too from your doctor.

Birth Planning After Trauma: Top Tips

At the end of this book we give some overall tips for birth planning in the context of anxiety. Here are some ideas, specifically if you are preparing for birth after trauma.

- If you feel able to, ensure those caring for you are aware of your experiences, how it has affected you and how you anticipate it might make childbirth and early parenthood difficult – it may be helpful to share this chapter with them. A partner, loved one or birth companion could support this if it feels too tricky.
- Consider the aspects of birth you feel most anxious about because of your trauma. Are there particular things you worry might trigger memories, strong emotions or feelings of dissociation? What might help enhance your sense of coping in those moments, discriminate then versus now and feel safe?
- What would people notice that would signal you need this help?
  What would you want them to say to you? To do? To give you or remind you of?
- Are there ways of staff communicating that would help you to feel more in control and held in their minds?
- For example, would you like early pain relief; support with breastfeeding or formula feeding; skin to skin or not?
- Are there specific ways to help you stay grounded, or differences you can be reminded to focus in on, e.g. having a special scent with you, music playing, staff explaining and seeking consent for each procedure; focusing on their tone of voice, shape of face, names of staff etc.
- Start to write down your ideas so you can bring these together in a clear plan nearer the end of your pregnancy, that can be shared with your care team and advocated by your birth partner or companion.
- Try to think through different scenarios (e.g. vaginal versus abdominal birth) with your birth partner and / or care team and what your preferences would be in each. This will help to build up your tolerance of uncertainty and enable you to take as flexible an approach as you can, e.g. during an abdominal birth you may prefer not to lie fully flat, you may want to have the curtain lowered in theatre so you can see your baby's birth or wear sunglasses if you worry the lights may be triggering for you.

When and How to Seek Professional Help for Traumatic Stress

If you believe you have PTSD or are feeling so affected by your experience that it is hard to function day to day, then it is likely you need more than this book, and will benefit from additional professional support. Try to talk to your midwife, doctor or other health professional at the earliest opportunity, so they can help you to access the support available to you in your area. In Chapter 1 we outlined the services which are currently available in England. These will differ slightly in Wales and Scotland, so talk to your midwife and doctor in the first instance for signposting.

National guidelines for clinical excellence in the treatment of PTSD (NICE, 2018) recommend either trauma-focused cognitive behaviour therapy (TF-CBT) or eye movement desensitisation and reprocessing (EMDR). Both these treatment options are considered 'high intensity' therapies, i.e. they involve (at least) weekly face-to-face (sometimes remote / virtual if preferred) contact with an appropriately trained and supervised therapist, usually for a minimum of 8–12 sessions.

Current evidence does not support the use of very brief trauma-focused interventions such as the 'three step Rewind technique' or one-off 'debriefing' sessions shortly after the event to review and relive the trauma for anyone experiencing PTSD. There is some evidence to suggest that a birth 'reflections' or birth review appointment with a birth professional can be useful in making sense of your experience if you have suffered a traumatic birth. For this to be helpful, you need to be with a clinician you trust, who can give the appropriate time and attention to hearing your experience and answering any questions in a setting that feels safe – i.e. preferably not the setting in which you were traumatised.

To Sum Up

- Birth- and maternity-related traumas are common, and are about how they were experienced rather than the degree of complications

- There are a range of symptoms that can follow after trauma, and it is helpful to know more about what these are
- Specific strategies can help reduce the intensity of trauma memories and the ongoing sense of threat and anxiety
- Working on your trauma memory, understanding the meaning of what happened and tackling avoidance and strategies can help you feel better and enjoy pregnancy or the postnatal period after trauma
- Sometimes professional help is needed, and this can be a very effective way to get more support to help you put these strategies in place

8

Anxiety About Pregnancy and Birth

In this chapter you will learn:

➤ What contributes to anxiety specific to pregnancy and birth ('pregnancy-specific anxiety') and what keeps it going

➤ The range of fears that mothers can experience during pregnancy, including the health of your baby, your bond with your baby, what birth will be like, your appearance during pregnancy or after birth, your parenting abilities and / or how life might change after birth

➤ How to recognise if this type of anxiety is creating problems for you

➤ Evidence-based techniques for tackling this type of anxiety

➤ Practical tips for talking to loved ones and health professionals about your anxiety, to ensure you are offered the right support

---

What Is Pregnancy-specific Anxiety?

There are many 'types' of anxiety, most of which share some common features, as you will see in the rest of this book. They can overlap with, but are not exactly the same as, pregnancy-specific anxiety, which is why we are focusing on it in this chapter. It often goes together with other anxiety problems, but research has shown that it is helpful to consider pregnancy-related anxiety as a distinct type of anxiety, characterised by *pregnancy-specific concerns.*

Most women will worry at some point about the health of their baby, how bonded they feel, how they will manage changes in their body, birth, or the upcoming tasks of parenthood and so on. Worrying in this way tends to be at its strongest in the first and third trimesters of pregnancy and is most common amongst first-time mums. This makes sense, as we get more worries when a situation is uncertain or unfamiliar, but it is not a problem that only affects first-time mothers. Whether this is your first pregnancy or fifth, every time is different, with unique challenges and uncertainties to navigate. On the contrary, difficult experiences in a previous pregnancy or birth may fuel worries about history repeating itself. Or sometimes simply hearing about others' difficult experiences can spark doubts and apprehension about how it will go for you.

Here are some common worries mums-to-be have told us about during their pregnancy:

What if my baby isn't healthy?
What if I do something to harm my baby?
What if my baby dies?
What if I can't bond with my baby?
What if I can't cope with looking after a newborn?
What if we don't have enough support?
Will I be able to cope with the pain of childbirth? Will my body be able to do it?
I can't cope with the uncertainty – I need to be sure my baby and I will be okay
What if I am abandoned and left alone during labour? What if no one listens to me?
What if my relationship can't manage the stress of parenting this baby?
What if my body is permanently changed by having a baby?
What if I lose my job? My friends?
What if my anxiety harms my baby?

For some mums-to-be, pregnancy-specific anxiety will be fleeting and easy to dismiss, but for others, anxiety like this can feel like it has hijacked life's driving seat and is well and truly in charge of their mind and behaviour. It may be problematic anxiety if it feels like you are consumed with worry, doubts or fearful thoughts for much of the day, and even though these feelings seem excessive and unreasonable, you struggle to turn your attention away from them. You might avoid situations for fear of triggering the thoughts (e.g. thinking or talking about pregnancy or birth; routine maternity appointments) or endure your day with intense distress. Significant pregnancy-specific anxiety is thought to affect a third of women in affluent countries, with possibly double that rate in low and middle income countries, where the conditions of birth and having children vary [1].

Severe Fear of Childbirth (Tokophobia)

One aspect of pregnancy-specific anxiety is a significant fear of childbirth, also known as tokophobia. Most women feel some degree of apprehension about birth. After all, this is a major life event which can feel uncertain and unpredictable and will be physically and emotionally challenging whether baby arrives vaginally or abdominally. However, for some women their anxiety is much more severe and disabling and significantly interferes with their quality of life. Recent estimates suggest 3.7% of women will suffer with a severe fear of childbirth, but many more of course will be experiencing mild to moderate anxieties about birth [2].

Themes highlighted by women and midwives include:

- A fear of not being able to cope with the pain of childbirth
- A fear of not knowing what will happen or being able to plan for the unpredictable
- A fear of harm or stress to the baby or oneself
- A fear of losing control
- Being abandoned or left alone
- Not having a voice in decision-making or having things 'done to' them [3].

At its most severe, tokophobia can leave some women avoiding pregnancy (or sex) altogether, enduring pregnancy with high levels of distress, or even terminating a pregnancy despite a desire to have a baby. Whether pregnant or not, avoidance of talking or thinking about birth is common, as well as feeling ashamed for fearing something that other people see as so 'natural'. If you are pregnant, such intense anxiety can make it feel impossible to enjoy pregnancy, can take away time from developing a bond with your baby or fully accessing all your choices around labour and birth. Difficulties sleeping, maintaining interest and motivation in your usual pleasures and low mood can follow. For some women, thoughts about giving birth may also trigger panic attacks or other health concerns – please see Chapter 5 on panic for further help if this is the case for you.

Tokophobia is usually separated by professionals into 'primary tokophobia', which is a longstanding fear often present since childhood, and 'secondary tokophobia', which is anxiety that has developed after a previous traumatic birth. In this second situation, the ideas in Chapter 7 on coping with trauma might also be helpful to look at. Primary tokophobia is often to do with hearing or seeing unhelpfully biased stories about childbirth at a sensitive age.

If you are experiencing primary or secondary tokophobia, it is important you are well supported – talk to your midwife as early as possible in your pregnancy about your fears, so they can help you access all the right support and make a birth plan that takes account of your and your baby's physical and mental health needs. If your anxiety is severe, you should also be referred for psychological support to a mental health specialist for pregnant women. Talking to someone who can answer your questions and understand your concerns in a supportive manner can help to reduce your anxiety. You should be offered evidence-based information so you can make informed choices about your birth. Some women with tokophobia will feel that an abdominal birth (C-section) is the best option for them as it is more predictable, and current national guidance states this should be offered when requested (NICE, 2019). The guidance also states that if an obstetrician is unwilling to carry out a C-section requested by a mother in these circumstances, then they must refer to another obstetrician who will. These conversations can help emphasise that you have choices. In any case, it is also helpful to work on managing your own thoughts and feelings about the birth.

> **KEY IDEA**
>
> *Some anxiety in pregnancy is normal. If it takes over and starts to disrupt day-to-day life then it may need your attention.*

Pregnancy-specific Anxiety

Rhea

Rhea was pregnant with her first baby. Although she very much wanted to be a mum, Rhea had put off trying to start a family with her husband for a long time, due to her anxiety about childbirth. As a little girl she remembers her mother and grandmother talking very graphically about their experiences of giving birth and how frightening it seemed to her. Her mother had spoken a number of times about how difficult Rhea's own birth had been and how Rhea would likely struggle too, given her 'small hips'.

Rhea had also had some difficult experiences in hospital in the past following a car accident, where she felt she wasn't listened to by doctors when she was in pain and was left without any pain relief for many hours. All of these experiences understandably left Rhea fearful that childbirth was dangerous, that she might not be able to cope with the pain, and that if she needed support she would be ignored.

Ultimately, she was terrified she and / or her baby might die. She wanted to aim for a vaginal birth but felt very little confidence her body was able to achieve this. Often images of her in hospital in agony alone would flash through her mind, especially if she saw anything birth related, e.g. an advert for 'One Born Every Minute' on TV or speaking with her midwife. She would feel sick and panicky, and would try hard to push the pictures out of her mind or avoid anything that might spark them off, but they still came back in abundance. She kept conversations brief at her maternity appointments and had yet to tell her midwife or husband just how scared she was feeling.

Rhea also found herself searching online for reassurance that her 'small hips' wouldn't cause problems for her. Often this meant she was presented with other people's difficult birth stories, which only made her feel more anxious. When several of her good friends had babies, she noticed she would either try to avoid discussions about their births or have a strong urge to ask for all the details of their experience that were difficult.

OVER TO YOU
Is Pregnancy-specific Anxiety a Problem for Me?

Recognising your pregnancy-related anxiety and how it is affecting you is important, because it is the first step to helping yourself feel better, asking for the support you need and giving yourself the best chance of feeling well when you meet your baby.

You may find it helpful to check the worries below which apply to you. Being specific about your fears can be very useful. We use the term 'worries', but these could be fears, thoughts, images etc. Please note this is not an exhaustive list. If your particular worry is not mentioned, feel free to add it at the end.

Pregnancy

I am worried about ...

Not bonding with my baby or not feeling the 'right way' about being pregnant
The physical changes to my body
The health of my baby
My baby dying
My anxiety harming my baby

Birth

I am worried about ...

Not coping with the pain of birth

Losing control in some way that would be humiliating, e.g. screaming or
   making too much noise, opening my bowels
Not being able to plan for every possibility – I can't cope with the uncertainty
   and unpredictability
Something bad happening to me (e.g. being injured or dying)
Something bad happening to my baby (e.g. being injured or dying)
My baby being born with a birth defect or unwell
Being abandoned or left alone
Being mistreated, 'having something done to me' or abused
Not being listened to
Not having control over decision-making
Not feeling love for my baby when they are born
Reliving past trauma

Parenthood

I am worried about ...

Not bonding with my baby
Not being able to cope with the demands of caring for a newborn (e.g. lack of
   sleep, baby crying)
Choosing the wrong name
My relationships suffering (e.g. with my partner, my friends, my other children,
   my family)
Not having enough support
My body not being the same
My life never being the same again

Other Worries ...

Remember, some anxiety is completely natural (and adaptive) in pregnancy, so many women will have had these thoughts at some point or another. It is only when anxiety becomes exaggerated and starts to disrupt
or interfere with your life that we would consider it a problem that needs
attention.

How Is Anxiety Affecting You?

- In the past few weeks have you been worrying about these things more often than not?
- Do you find it hard to stop, control or turn your attention away from your worries and anxious thoughts?
- How do these thoughts make you feel? E.g. fearful, guilty, ashamed, angry, panicked (it could be more than one)
- Does your anxiety stop you from doing things you would like to do? Or make day-to-day tasks more difficult than usual? What sorts of things? E.g. appointments, sleep, planning / buying things for your baby, talking / thinking about pregnancy / baby, seeing friends, watching TV etc.
- Does the anxiety pull you into taking excessive precautions to feel safer? E.g. seeking reassurance, preparing for the worst, repeatedly checking or over-researching etc.
- How does it leave you feeling physically? E.g. tense, nauseous, tired, restless, unable to relax or concentrate etc.

Understanding Pregnancy-specific Anxiety

Why Have I Developed Pregnancy-specific Anxiety?

Everyone has a combination of vulnerabilities and strengths, and research highlights a number of different factors which are associated with anxiety in pregnancy – biological, environmental and psychological. These include (but are not limited to) the physical changes and demands of pregnancy, your previous life experiences (including those around conception and / or other pregnancies) and how these might shape your expectations of your pregnancy, birth and motherhood, your self-esteem, your current circumstances and the support available to you (or not). Let's look at some of these in more detail.

Evolution and Changes in Threat Sensitivity during Pregnancy

Anxiety and evolution are inextricably linked. We know that anxiety is a key adaptive feeling that has enabled the survival of our species and is a basic emotion common to mammals. It readies you to protect yourself through what is commonly called our 'fight, flight or freeze' response. It makes sense then that the part of your nervous system that signals danger might become more sensitive or alert when you are pregnant, so that you and your baby have the best chance of survival. Experimental research backs up the idea that it is adaptive to be more cautious and more alert to danger at this time. For example, one study has shown that pregnant women show increased attention to threatening cues (e.g. pictures of fearful versus neutral faces) compared to non-pregnant women.

The Physical Demands of Pregnancy

Many physiological changes happen in pregnancy to nurture your developing baby and prepare your body for birth. Your hormone levels; the efficiency of your heart, lungs and gut; flexibility of your joints and muscles; and your body temperature all change. No organ in the body is unaffected. The consequences of some of these changes might be expected, e.g. feeling or being sick; increased fatigue and appetite, gaining weight and changing shape; an aching back or joints; increased urgency and frequency to pee; changes in our breast size, hair and skin, and so on. Others might be less expected, e.g. varicose veins, skin breakouts, constipation and acid reflux, insomnia, restless legs, gasping for breath when you've only climbed a few stairs, bigger feet and darker nipples! In addition, some sensations which you may have hoped to enjoy (e.g. feeling your baby move) can trigger worry about what that might mean about the health of your baby or you as a mother.

Many of these physical changes will make it harder for you to regulate your emotions, and consequently you may find yourself feeling more easily upset or overwhelmed – after all, if you're feeling tired, in pain, sick and / or hungry, managing your usual daily tasks such as a busy journey, a demanding work meeting or the needs of young children will be understandably much more difficult. Your usual resources are depleted by the task of growing a baby and your usual ways of coping with life's challenges or relaxing (e.g. having a drink, going for a long run) might be harder to access because of the physical changes you are experiencing.

Pregnancy might also exacerbate underlying physical health issues you already experience, e.g. thyroid dysfunction, heart disease or result in the development of new complications specific to pregnancy, e.g. gestational diabetes, hyperemesis, pelvic pain (also known as symphysis pubis dysfunction, (SPD)). Health professionals might (unhelpfully) talk about these physical complications as deeming your pregnancy 'high risk' or 'not normal'. Note that this is a really broad category! All of this is bound to be stressful and fuel worry.

Having Had Anxiety or Other Problems in the Past

Research has shown that a family, or more specifically, a personal history of mental health difficulties does raise the risk for antenatal anxiety. This makes sense, as most difficulties emerge from a combination of vulnerabilities and stress, and it is a stressful time. However, it is also important to note that many, and possibly most, women with a previous personal or family history of mental health difficulties stay well during pregnancy and beyond. Although we can't change the past or our genetics, there is also much that you can do. If you can, seeking out good-quality support during pregnancy, being physically active and eating well are good basics to aim for. Having good problem-solving skills, a sense of agency and positive self-esteem have all been shown to be protective. There are lots of tips and exercises in earlier chapters that can help with many of these. Working on these things alongside actively tackling the beliefs and behaviours that keep your anxiety going give you a very good chance of staying well.

Your Journey to Pregnancy

It makes sense that the road you have travelled to be pregnant will play a role in how you feel now. For some, falling pregnant happens quickly, while for others trying to conceive can be a long and painful road. Fertility issues are often described as a 'silent struggle' and still, sadly, often feel like a taboo topic, although one in seven couples will have difficulties conceiving. A pregnancy may be planned or unplanned, wanted or unwanted, or it's possible to have mixed and ambivalent feelings. Some people will have experienced ectopic pregnancies and / or miscarriage(s), for others, complications will mean they have had to come to the unbearably hard decision to end a much-wanted pregnancy.

Research shows that pregnancy-specific anxiety, understandably, is particularly heightened for women who:

- Have experienced a previous pregnancy loss, stillbirth or termination
- Have a pregnancy which was unexpected or undesired
- Have had a previous birth experience which was traumatic
- Only have a short interval following a miscarriage before a subsequent pregnancy

It is of course possible to feel anxious in the absence of these experiences. Sometimes people become pregnant unexpectedly, or very quickly, and can feel terribly unprepared. The journey is very individual, but there are always factors that make sense of your experience. Being understanding of yourself can be helpful in moving forward.

Earlier Life Experiences

Our life experiences (or perhaps more importantly the meaning we attach to these experiences) shape our beliefs and assumptions about ourselves, the world around us and our future. Some experiences will impact us more than others, and some will be particularly pertinent to understanding the ideas and expectations we have of pregnancy, birth and parenthood. For example, studies have shown that the quality of our relationship with our own parents can have a significant effect on how anxious or low we feel during pregnancy.

If you have not had a good caregiving experience as a child yourself, this can naturally make the idea of being a parent more challenging or hard to cope with. Being pregnant may remind you of how difficult things were for you in the past and you might worry about history repeating itself and becoming a version of your own parent(s). Remember that you are not them; you are a unique individual and that you are taking responsible steps to work on your anxiety and understand how to minimise the impact on you and your baby.

These memories might mean you view yourself as less competent / able to cope, or put pressure on yourself to do things differently. Or you might simply struggle to connect with the idea of being a mother at all. Our section on building a relationship with your baby in Chapter 9 can help with things to try if you are experiencing this, as well as some of the resources listed at the end of this book.

For other women, past abuse (either as a child or adult) or other distressing experiences (e.g. bereavements, difficult medical or surgical experiences) may have a considerable impact on their experience and expectations of pregnancy and birth. They may worry about being mistreated again, find aspects of pregnancy or the prospect of birth very triggering or experience a heightened sense of threat around something bad happening to them again. If this is the case for you, do take a look at Chapter 7 on trauma for more ideas on how to manage the impact of these experiences during pregnancy. There are also more resources at the end of this book if you want to work more deeply on low self-esteem and childhood trauma.

Current Circumstances

Life is full of potential stressors. Many studies have shown that adverse events during pregnancy can contribute to psychological distress. These might include the death or illness of a relative, a relationship breakdown, work stress, financial worries or moving or renovating your home. How stressful these experiences are will depend in part on the meaning we attach to them (as we highlighted in the introduction) and our belief in our capacity to cope and adapt. The resources around us, specifically social support, has an important role to play in reducing the negative impact of these events. Women who experience stressful life events but have good social support in place are much less likely to suffer from lasting emotional distress than women without an available support network.

You may be experiencing domestic violence or abuse including physical, sexual, emotional abuse or controlling behaviour. Pregnancy is a time of increased risk for these things. Please see our resources section at the end of this book for where to seek help, including urgently if you feel unsafe. Abuse of any kind can contribute to symptoms of anxiety and depression and is also more frequent in circumstances of greater environmental stress such as pandemics. These huge global events change behaviour in important ways. The section towards the end of this book on the impact of the Covid-19 pandemic has more information on how the situation around you may impact on anxiety in various ways and how to navigate it.

Messages from Others

In the previous example we saw how Rhea was impacted by the conversations in her family about birth and how this linked to the anxiety she was experiencing now she was pregnant. They may not always be obvious, but other people's ideas and assumptions about pregnancy and birth are all around us – from the stories within our own families and friendship groups, through the ideals that exist in our specific culture about the roles and responsibilities of motherhood, to the ways pregnancy and birth are portrayed in the media and wider society.

When you are pregnant, you are confronted with lists of rules. 'Advice' about what we can and can't do as women to make sure we keep our baby healthy and safe and the 'risks' we and our baby face can also feel like they bombard us at every turn – what to eat, how to sleep, what activities we 'should' and 'shouldn't' do. It's no wonder women can end up feeling pressure, scrutinised and hypervigilant for doing the 'wrong' thing. Women are left in an exhausting struggle between heightened responsibility and not being able to control all the variables. Research shows that reasoning about risk in pregnancy is notoriously challenging, not just for women but for health professionals too – what is 'dangerous' versus 'safe'; 'reckless' versus 'responsible'.

Too often the messages and warnings we get about what to avoid are driven by fear of doing harm rather than an evidence base supporting actual danger – a 'better safe than sorry', all or nothing approach which trumps a balanced evaluation of risks and benefits for the individual mother and baby. It can be very skewed. For example, women are routinely warned not to eat raw seafood such as sushi due to worry about the possible risk of illness, but the actual risk of falling ill from seafood is one in two million servings, which is actually less common when compared to other widely consumed foods! The consequence of all this is women can end up feeling like they must strive to meet an impossible standard of zero risk in pregnancy, often at the cost of taking care of their own needs. An approach which not surprisingly fuels anxiety.

KEY IDEA

Many factors understandably increase anxiety in pregnancy. Anxiety is not your fault, but you can take responsibility for tackling it.

Understanding What Is Keeping You Stuck: What Keeps Pregnancy-specific Anxiety Going?

Your Specific Beliefs About Pregnancy, Birth and Parenting

Problems with anxiety persist not because of the situation itself but the *meaning* we attach or *interpretation* we give a certain event. This helps us to understand why the same event (e.g. pregnancy or anticipation of birth) might affect people differently and lead some people to worry more than others. In Chapter 1 we described the important role your own ideas about likelihood, awfulness, coping and rescue play in anxiety.

OVER TO YOU

Identifying Your Specific Beliefs about Pregnancy, Birth and Parenting

Step 1: Catching Your Thoughts

When you are confronted with a particular situation linked to your fears (it could be an activity, a body sensation, thought, image or memory) quick thoughts or images can be triggered. They are usually automatic or uninvited – i.e. outside of conscious control and appear even if you don't want them to, or you might anticipate them (because we know a particular situation is often difficult).

Here are some examples of Rhea's quick thoughts:

Situation	Thought / Image	Feelings
Watching TV, advert for a series based on maternity comes on	Image of being alone and in agony	Panicked, sick
Talking to a midwife	I can't cope with talking about this	Tense
Coffee with a friend and her new baby	She is petite and her birth sounds terrible, so I am bound to have a bad birth too. Memory of mum talking about my hips	Fearful

Are there particular situations you have noticed which tend to be particularly stressful for you or trigger a lot of anxiety? For example, certain conversations, activities, feeling certain body sensations or baby movements etc. Try to think of a recent time when you were in one of these situations and really bothered by your anxiety about pregnancy, birth or parenthood.

Getting a specific example of the problem clear in your mind will help you to catch any quick thoughts that pop up. Go back in your head to that time and try to bring as much detail to mind as possible of the situation you were in:

- Where were you?
- Who were you with?
- What was happening?

Once you have set the scene, try to identify the first sign of 'trouble', i.e. that anxiety was on the rise:

- What were you feeling? Tense, nervous, on edge? Fearful or panicked?
- Did you notice any particular thoughts, images or memories going through your mind?
- If that is tricky to remember, ask yourself what you were feeling most nervous, fearful or anxious about? What did your anxiety say might happen or was happening?

Situation	Quick thoughts / images	Feelings

Step 2: Working Out Your Underlying Fears

These quick thoughts provide us with an opportunity to understand the key underlying fears which drive your pregnancy-specific anxiety. Let's see how this worked for Rhea:

Rhea

What is the quick thought bothering you?	Image of being alone and in agony
If this were true what would this mean? What would be the worst thing about that for you?	Birth is going to be horrendous It will be unbearably painful
What would that say about you? How well would you cope? How well will others support you?	I'm a failure as a woman I won't be able to They won't listen to me or help me. I will just be ignored
Ultimately what is the very worst thing that you think will happen as a consequence?	My baby or I will die

Try to freeze frame a moment that the anxiety struck and ask yourself the same questions as Rhea to see if you can uncover the fears underlying your anxiety:

What is the quick thought bothering you?	
What do you think will happen? What would make this so awful for you? What would that say about you? What would that mean for your future? Ultimately what is the very worst thing that you think will happen as a consequence?	

OVER TO YOU
What Habits Do You Notice in Your Thinking?

We spoke about common thinking styles in anxiety in Chapter 1 – have you spotted any habits in your thinking? What effect do they have on how you view a situation in pregnancy or how you end up feeling? It can help to start to keep a lookout for these habits and notice them in action so you can remind yourself of how they trip you up.

Catastrophising (thinking the worse)	
All or nothing thinking	
Shoulds and musts	
Rumination / post-mortems on situations	
Worry – what ifs	
Magical thinking	
Self-attacking	
Using feelings as evidence (emotional reasoning)	

What You Do to Try to Feel Better and How It Might Make Things Worse: Safety-seeking Behaviours and Avoidance

In the 'What Is Anxiety' section in Chapter 1 we also spoke about how the interpretations we make in any given situation will drive understandable reactions that are intended to help us 'seek safety' but usually keep our sense of threat and anxiety going. In a sense the solutions we are turning to in order to feel better become the problem. These might be behaviours, our focus of attention, or processes happening inside our head (e.g. rumination or trying to suppress anxious thoughts). If you are anxious about some aspect of pregnancy or birth, it is very likely some (or all) of the following reactions are at play.

Avoidance

Avoidance is one of the most common ways to deal with anxiety. After all, it makes rational sense to avoid the things we fear may harm us or cause us distress. Like Rhea, you may be avoiding situations which trigger anxious thoughts, images and feelings around pregnancy, birth or parenting (e.g. antenatal appointments and classes, looking in the mirror, TV programmes, reading anything related to pregnancy or birth or perhaps trying to conceal your bump to avoid questions about the pregnancy); trying to suppress or 'neutralise' these thoughts in some way (e.g. by frantically distracting yourself, trying to push the thoughts out of your mind or 'thinking positively') or avoiding situations which you worry might be risky for you and your baby (e.g. eating or drinking certain foods, going outside for fear of traffic fumes, coming into contact with dog, cat or fox faeces). Sometimes avoidance might also follow from what is known as superstitious or 'magical' thinking. In some cultures, there is often a strong message that saying, doing or thinking certain things will be unlucky, 'jinx' things or 'tempt fate'. The same can be true around pregnancy and / or birth, e.g. 'Something bad is bound to happen to my baby if I pack my hospital bag or start getting ready.'

Avoidance can feel helpful in the short term – your anxiety will usually lessen when you aren't confronted with the situation, but it can be very limiting, damage your confidence and stop you from putting your fears to the test. It might also mean you end up with less support at a time when having people around you is crucial. Repeated avoidance means that the next time you encounter the same situation you will feel all the more overwhelmed and afraid. By avoiding situations, you also buy into the idea that you (or your baby) are in danger, either now or in the future, which naturally fuels your fears all the more, and so an unpleasant vicious cycle develops. Avoidance can also trigger a host of other unwanted emotions, e.g. guilt, shame, frustration, so it is never a good long-term solution to tackling pregnancy-specific anxiety.

What You Pay Attention To: Heightened Awareness to Internal and External Threats

When you are anxious, you may also notice that you feel more alert and sensitive to what is happening in your surroundings or in your body. This is a normal reaction, as it is your brain's way of protecting you from harm. It is also a particularly common experience after trauma (see Chapter 7 on this for more information). You might feel like your mind is constantly looking for signs of trouble or ways to escape from harm's way. Usually, the focus of your attention will fall on things that have been flagged in your mind as a potential threat – your mind 'zooms in' on what feels important. For example, during the Covid-19 pandemic, a very strong public health message was sent out about the importance of keeping 2 metres apart to reduce the risk of spreading infection. Before the pandemic, you probably wouldn't have routinely paid that much attention to how close other people were to you, but during the height of the pandemic this was flagged as a threat – consequently what did you tend to notice or monitor when you were around other people?

In pregnancy, you might focus in on what is going on around you if that feels worrying to you, but very often your attention will focus on what is happening inside your body. For example, if you are feeling very fearful of miscarriage, you might notice your attention 'zooming in' on unusual sensations or constantly monitoring how much your baby is moving. Sometimes this is reinforced by maternity guidelines such as monitoring your baby's movements. Whilst getting to know your baby's movements is recommended as a way to assure that they are well, many mums find this an added source of stress and anxiety – how much movement is enough? How do I monitor them? What if I miss a reduction in movement? It might feel all consuming, with constant doubts about whether they are okay. So what is designed to try and help reassure mums can become a hindrance, as it amplifies feelings of uncertainty and danger and possibly means noticing or bringing on new sensations, which then fuel more worry. We will come back to this specific dilemma below.

Seeking Certainty

Anxiety can set you the impossible task of being completely sure of something before it allows you to relax or make a decision on what to do next. For example, it might say 'Can you be absolutely certain this is the best, safest car seat out there?'; 'Are you 100% confident you felt your baby move in the right way just then?'; 'Are you sure you are bonding with your baby enough?'. Or it might say 'You need to know everything there is to know about birth in order for things to go well.' And when it asks these questions, how do you tend to feel? Trying to achieve certainty is a natural way to respond when faced with doubt. For example, you might repeatedly ask for reassurance from a loved one or medical professional or seek it through online research or in books. The riskier a situation feels the higher the level of certainty anxiety demands. The difficulty is, reassurance seeking in this way doesn't tend to work long term or even in the short term, because 100% certainty is impossible. Uncertainty is a part of life. An alternative to seeking certainty is to accept a little bit of uncertainty and to build your tolerance of it. We will show you some ways to do this here and in Chapter 2 on worry.

Your Circumstances and Support Network

A final area to think about in understanding what might be maintaining your anxiety in the here and now are your current circumstances. Are there aspects of your life at the moment which are adding to your overall levels of stress? Ways you feel unsupported or isolated from those around you – either loved ones or health professionals? Ways your pregnancy is proving physically or logistically challenging, e.g. managing antenatal appointments around work commitments or caring for other children. These aren't always things that are straightforward to change but considering them might help make sense of your experience and decide whether there are ways to problem solve in order to reduce your stress and increase your support network.

Bringing It All Together: A Vicious 'Flower' of Pregnancy-specific Anxiety

Putting all these things together, there are a number of factors in the present that can make fearful thoughts about pregnancy, birth and parenthood feel all the more believable and harder to ignore. They operate as simultaneous vicious circles which we call a 'vicious flower' of pregnancy-specific anxiety. Above the flower we also take into account past experiences and underlying ideas about yourself and the world which might mean pregnancy, birth and parenthood (or situations associated with them) are viewed through a particularly anxious lens.

You can see Rhea's vicious flower below:

Vicious flower of Rhea's anxiety

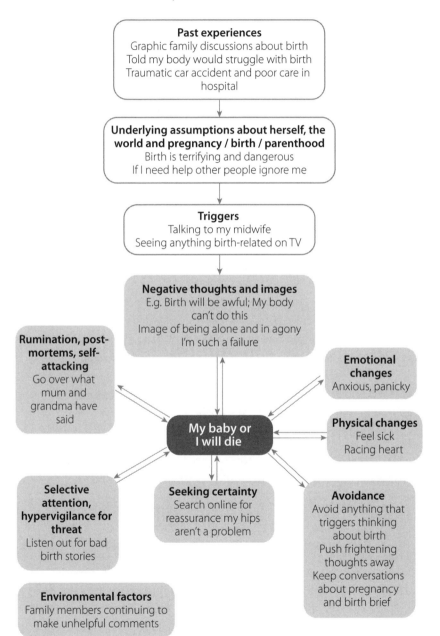

OVER TO YOU

Mapping Your Own Vicious Flower

Look back over the previous exercises. What past experiences and underlying ideas seem relevant to your anxiety in the here and now?

Take the specific example you thought about above and make a note of the negative thoughts (and / or images) you spotted and the ultimate feared consequence you unpacked. Now consider:

- What emotion was triggered in that situation? You may have felt anxious, afraid, panicked, uncomfortable, worried or perhaps some other feeling such as low, angry or disgusted. Jot down everything that applies. There is no right or wrong answer.
- What did you do to try to deal with what was happening?
- What did you do to try to manage the discomfort or fear or simply stop something bad from happening?
- Consider the things you did physically (e.g. online research, asking for reassurance, avoiding situations etc.) as well as in your mind (e.g. trying to suppress or argue back against the thoughts and images, plan out every possible scenario or what you might need to do if your fear was true).
- Where was the focus of your attention? Were you concentrating on anything in particular, e.g. a body sensation, a facial expression or were you focused on the churning worry in your mind? Were you 'scanning for danger' or 'looking for signs of trouble' in some way?
- Was there anything else you did to try and deal with the anxiety?

Next, have a think about the consequences of the ways you tried to cope on your central beliefs about pregnancy, birth and parenthood:

- Do you think they make these ideas seem more or less believable?
- Do these ways of coping 'buy into' your fears?
- What message do they give you about how safe you and your baby are and / or how capable and competent you are?

It is worth going through a few different examples to see if the anxiety always works in the same way for you. If you have fears about aspects of birth as well as pregnancy, it may be worth drawing out a separate vicious flower for both, to see if the factors maintaining your anxiety about each issue are the same or different.

Vicious flower of pregnancy-specific anxiety

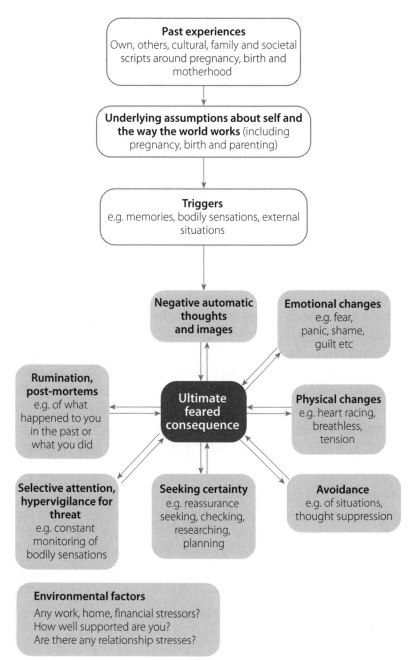

Moving Forward: Breaking Free from Excessive Anxiety about Pregnancy and / or Birth

Finding an Alternative Explanation for What Is Going On: Theory A versus Theory B

Often, up until now, the key meanings which drive your anxiety (the ideas in the centre of your vicious flower) will have been accepted as fact, e.g. 'Birth is more dangerous for me'; 'My baby will die'; 'I won't love my baby'; 'I won't cope with the demands of parenting'; 'No-one can be trusted to keep my baby and I safe'; and life has been lived accordingly. But what if you treat these not as facts but ideas that can be examined; and even if your concerns have *some* evidence to support them (which can often be the case), what if there is another more helpful way of looking at the problem?

Anxiety has convinced you that the problem you need to address is that something bad or dangerous *will* happen during pregnancy, birth or parenthood. It might convince you that this will be your fault and that it is your responsibility to do something about it, that you're incapable of managing these challenges or that you are a bad mother. But what if the problem that needs solving is not danger but the *worry (perhaps even terror)* about something dangerous or terrible happening? Being stuck in constant fear is probably already hurting you and stopping you from having the pregnancy you hoped for – what if *this* is the real issue that needs to be tackled now?

We call these two possibilities or ways of thinking about the problem that you need to solve, Theory A (the problem is danger) and Theory B (the problem is *worry* about danger) and we consider them two competing explanations. In this sense they cannot both be true at the same time and they will have very different implications for what you do to solve the things you are struggling with.

Let's look at how this might work for Rhea as an example.

For Rhea, her anxiety tells her that the problem is 'Birth will be dangerous for you, no-one will help you and you won't be able to cope' (Theory A).

An alternative way of looking at Rhea's difficulties might be: 'Because of what you have heard from others and your experiences in hospital in the past, you understandably worry that birth will be dangerous and difficult for you and lack confidence in other people's support and your ability to cope' (Theory B).

So, Theory B is that the problem *itself* is one of anxiety and all the things it tries to get you to do to stay safe / avoid the worst from happening. It is saying that you are overestimating the likelihood of danger and underestimating your ability to cope if things are difficult. This is very different from saying the problem is danger itself. It is really important to remember that the problem is *understandable* worry and takes into account the impact of previous life experiences.

Some other possible ways of looking at Theories A and B which others have found helpful are:

Theory A	Theory B
My body can't do this (competence problem)	I lack confidence in my body to do this (confidence problem)
I feel uncertain, so disaster must lie ahead (a disaster problem)	I am understandably struggling to tolerate uncertainty (tolerance of uncertainty problem)

OVER TO YOU
Your Theory A versus Theory B

My Theory A (What anxiety *says* the problem is – i.e. what is in the centre of your vicious flower):

My Theory B (My alternative way of looking at this – how anxiety *is* the problem):

Examining the Evidence for Theory A and Theory B

In order to work out which of these theories best fits your experience, both now and in the past, it is important to take a look at the evidence you have so far. Based on what we have previously discussed, you might already have an idea of the sorts of things which make Theory A feel more believable, e.g. things which have happened to you, to others, the opinions of others, how others have behaved towards you, your emotions and physical feelings in the moment and so on. It is important to examine the evidence for both theories as objectively as possible, and not accept anything ambiguous or subjective – much like you would do if you were arguing a case in court. The standard of evidence must be high – is it factual and reliable? Here is an example from a second-time Mum.

Theory A	Theory B
The problem is …	The problem is …
I am incapable of dealing with the demands of a second baby and my life will fall apart	*My past experiences have left me very fearful about life with a second baby and mean I underestimate my capacity to cope*
Why do I believe this?	
I really struggled after my first baby *I have seen other women struggling with more than one child*	*Life was hard last time but did not fall apart* *My son is healthy and happy and I enjoy him now* *I know that however difficult things felt then they did pass and got better* *People often tell me I think the worst of myself and underestimate my abilities* *I know things now I didn't know then about what helps me feel less overwhelmed* *There are people who can support us and I know who to ask for help* *There have been ways to continue what is important to me even with a baby, e.g. …* *Situations that are unpredictable and unfamiliar often make me anxious*

Here is Rhea's example:

Theory A	Theory B
The problem is ...	The problem is ...
Birth will be dangerous for me. No-one will help me and I won't be able to cope	*Because of what I have heard from others and my experiences in hospital in the past I understandably worry that birth will be dangerous and difficult for me and underestimate other people's support and my ability to cope*
Why do I believe this?	
Frightening conversations between Mum and Ammi *Mum telling me I will struggle because of 'small hips'* *Difficult experience in hospital after the crash* *Friends have had difficult births*	*I think I am probably worrying more than the average person about birth* *The obstetrician told me the size of my hips is not an issue for birth* *Professionals so far have been attentive* *I often struggle with situations which are uncertain and new*

OVER TO YOU
Evidence for Theory A and Theory B

Theory A	Theory B
The problem is ...	The problem is ...
Why do I believe this?	

Implications for Theories A and B: What Do You Need to Do to Solve the Problem? And What Does This Mean for the Remainder of the Pregnancy and Beyond?

If you took Theory A as a definitive statement of your problem and believed it wholeheartedly (which is likely how it has been defined up until now) what would that mean you needed to do? What are the rules you would need to follow? And if you keep following these rules, what will that mean for your pregnancy and your future life? And how about Theory B – what would Theory B say you needed to do?

Let's look at what Rhea would need to do if her Theory A was true, and then if her Theory B were true:

Rhea

Theory A	Theory B
The problem is …	The problem is …
Birth will be dangerous for me. No one will help me and I won't be able to cope	*Because of what I have heard from others and my experiences in hospital in the past, I understandably worry that birth will be dangerous and difficult for me and lack confidence in other people's support and my ability to cope*
What do I need to do if I treat this idea as true?	
Review the evidence that I am at risk – go over conversations and past experiences *Look for reassurance about my hips on Google* *Avoid anything that triggers thoughts of birth*	*Get reliable information on my hips and my personal risks for birth* *Talk to the medical team about what I need to feel supported and to understand my options fully for birth* *Talk to my husband and friends about how I am feeling so they can support me better* *Widen my lens around birth stories – notice positive experiences as well as the more difficult ones* *Evaluate the idea I can't cope with pain*
What happens if I carry on doing these things?	
Feel more and more anxious and isolated *Birth seems more and more likely to be awful* *Feel even more like a failure*	*Hopefully feel less anxious and better able to cope* *Feel more confident in the support around me and my ability to have a positive birth experience*

OVER TO YOU
Implications for Theory A and Theory B

Hopefully, in looking through Rhea's example, you will have begun to see there is an alternative way of understanding what you are experiencing. You don't have to fully believe Theory B yet – the more important thing is to be open to considering it as a possibility and be willing to put each theory to the test so you can work out which approach helps reduce your anxiety best.

Solving an anxiety problem usually means doing the opposite of what you would do if you were in actual danger. So, overcoming your anxiety means tackling all the things which amplify your fears, i.e. the thinking habits and ways of coping we outlined earlier. So, trying to approach rather than avoid tricky situations, accepting uncertainty rather than striving for certainty, connecting rather than withdrawing from those around you, problem-solving rather than churning worry over, building up your confidence in yourself as well as bringing compassion rather than criticism to how you are feeling.

Theory A	Theory B
The problem is …	The problem is …
What do I need to do if I treat this idea as true?	
What happens if I carry on doing these things?	

Moving Forward: Setting Goals and Putting Theory into Practice

Completing the Theory A and Theory B table will hopefully have helped you begin to think about what steps you might need to take to tackle your anxiety. It might involve working on some of the unhelpful thinking patterns you have spotted but also (and perhaps more importantly) changing what you do when you feel anxious or notice yourself starting to worry. The last two sections of Theory B are essentially an action plan of what to aim for and how things will hopefully be better if you stick with it.

Now is a good time to start thinking about what you would like to be different. How would you like things to improve in the short and longer term? How would you know if things were moving in the right direction? What behaviours would you like to try and change or eliminate altogether? Are there things you would like to be doing which you are not doing now? Try to make your goals as specific as possible and something that is easy to measure and observe. 'I want to feel less scared about giving birth' is an understandable goal, but how would you know if this was happening? What would you be doing more or less of that you aren't doing now? What would other people notice?

Rhea's goals
Stop Googling e.g. 'hip width birth death'
Talk to the medical team about my actual risks with my hips and my birth options
Talk to my husband and friends about how I am feeling
Find some positive birth stories to balance the negative
Get more comfortable with uncertainty
Start planning what to buy for the baby
Download baby buddy app

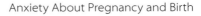

OVER TO YOU
What Are Your Specific Goals

Moving Forward: Making Changes Where You Can

In this section we will talk about some of the specific steps you can take to begin to tackle your anxiety in pregnancy. This will include:

- Taking reasonable steps to be well informed, to help you feel more empowered and in control
- Building up a realistic view of risk, your capacity to cope and the resources available to support you
- Developing ways to tolerate and accept uncertainty
- Reducing unhelpful ways of coping such as avoidance, worry, tuning into danger, checking and reassurance seeking
- Building a more compassionate (rather than critical) approach to your struggles

Gathering Reliable Information to Help You Evaluate Your Fears

If this is your first pregnancy (or even if not), some of your fear may be understandably linked to what is unfamiliar and unknown. Research shows that good-quality education about pregnancy, birth and early parenting can help reduce anxiety, as it reduces unpredictability, offers alternative explanations for things that may have been worrying you (e.g. unexplained body sensations) and allows you to consider what you may need to feel well supported and retain a sense of control (e.g. what birth options you would prefer, what support might be helpful to you after birth). Reliable information will also help you fairly evaluate your personal risks and compare these to your 'felt sense' which can be a bit off – i.e. you might fear that a particular complication or difficulty is highly likely for you, but knowing the actual likelihood can help you consider if your feelings are an overestimate or not (and consequently how much attention they deserve). It should also give you an opportunity to 'widen' your lens around the focus of your fears so you can access balanced, evidence-based information rather than only negative anecdotes.

Be Specific

Try and focus on the specific questions you would find helpful to have answered before you access further information, so you can target your anxiety efficiently and effectively. Think about what you need to know / understand better to feel less anxious. For example, Rhea wanted to know 'Are my hips below average size?'; 'Does hip size predict birth outcomes?'; 'What are my pain relief options during birth and how can I access them?'; 'Will I be left alone at any point during labour?'. Of course, you may have different questions at different points during pregnancy. At whatever stage, the key is to try and keep these questions focused and specific.

Go to Reliable Sources

Consider your source of information carefully. Try to avoid general web searches, as the quality and accuracy of information your searches return cannot be guaranteed. Relying on one or two friends or family may also be unhelpful, as their experience is limited to themselves and they may have particular views which aren't supported by the available evidence. It is better to try and speak with your health care provider if you can in the first instance – i.e. your midwife, obstetrician etc., as they should have access to up-to-date evidence. Other good sources of information include the baby buddy app (www.bestbeginnings.org.uk/baby-buddy), and the National Institute for Health and Care Excellence (www.evidence.nhs.uk) or you may want to sign up to antenatal classes (in the UK, the NHS offers free-to-access classes, so ask your midwife about these).

If you've been avoiding things like this, you may find it helpful to set it up as an experiment, to help you to plan more specifically where to start, what you will do, who you will speak to and why. Having someone supportive with you can also be helpful, as taking in and remembering information when you are anxious is more difficult. If this isn't possible, consider what might help you to keep track of what is being said or what you are reading, e.g. having regular pauses, writing down or recording key information in some way and so on.

Remember the aim here is not to feel absolutely certain, as that is impossible – there is risk in pregnancy and birth in the same way as there is risk in most aspects of life (see 'Accepting Some Uncertainty'). What you are aiming for is to have more concrete information to help you evaluate whether your fears are fair – i.e. are you overestimating the likelihood and awfulness of something happening and / or underestimating your ability to cope and that of those around you to help? If you notice yourself needing to return to information repeatedly to try and feel certain, then information gathering may be functioning more as reassurance seeking and maintaining your anxiety. If this is the case, it will be helpful to experiment with trying to stop repeatedly checking or asking for reassurance (or delaying acting on the urge) – see the following for more tips on this and Chapter 3 on dealing with unwanted intrusive thoughts.

OVER TO YOU
Evaluating Your Fears

> What specific questions do you have about pregnancy, birth or early parenthood which link to your anxiety?
> Who could help you to answer these questions?
> What would help you to hold onto what is said?

> Think ahead to what you would like to know about the next stage (next trimester, birth, labour, hospital, early postnatal period).

Testing Things Out: Experimenting with Doing Things Differently

'Behavioural experiments' are a key tool to help tackle anxiety and something we revisit regularly through the chapters of this book. They are ways of testing out anxious predictions and finding out what happens if we change the way we respond to feeling anxious, e.g. reducing avoidance, checking, reassurance seeking and so on. Working through the Theory A versus Theory B framework in this chapter may have given you some ideas of ways you might need to experiment with doing things differently to begin to tackle your anxiety about pregnancy, birth or early parenthood. For Rhea, this included experiments to see what happens when she reduced reassurance seeking, talked to her friends and boss about her pregnancy (rather than avoiding them) and allowed herself to look in the mirror.

Here is an example of one of Rhea's experiments:

Complete before the experiment		Complete after the experiment	
What am I testing out?	My specific predictions and how much I believe them	Did my predictions come true?	What did I find out?
The next time I have the urge to ask Rob if everything will be okay or if he still finds me attractive, I will do my best not to, and try and turn my attention onto something else	I will feel unbearably anxious (95%)	No. I felt very anxious initially and found it hard to concentrate as my mind kept bouncing back to the idea everything will go wrong, but within a few minutes the anxiety and urge did start to ease	I can cope without having immediate reassurance The anxiety and urge passes Rob can support me in other ways, e.g. giving me a hug etc. I could try again like this the next time the urge pops up
	I won't be able to resist the urge and will have to ask him (80%)	I didn't ask him (although I told him I was doing my best not to)	

The idea is to deliberately experiment with doing things differently, in order to put a specific fear to the test (usually something driven by Theory A). You want this to be as fair a test as possible, so it is important to try and let go of any of the usual precautions you might take when you are anxious, so that you can find out how the world really works. Try to start with a situation that feels manageable but still anxiety provoking and work up to more challenging tasks to help build your confidence.

Other pregnancy-specific anxious thoughts which might be helpfully tackled with a behavioural experiment include:

1. If I think or talk about pregnancy, birth or parenting I will become overwhelmed (reduce avoidance to check out fears about capacity to cope with feeling anxious)
2. If I do X then something bad will happen to my baby (check out magical thinking)

3. If I talk to people about how I am feeling I will be ignored (check out fears around support)
4. If I don't do X I will feel unbearably anxious and won't be able to function (check out fears of dropping usual precautions and ways of coping)

OVER TO YOU
Testing Things Out

Are there specific predictions you could put to the test using a behavioural experiment? Try to link these to your goals and use the framework below to help you.

If you are not sure where to start, then think about what you are not doing or what you are avoiding, and pick one of those things. Plan doing it 'normally' without taking precautions.

Complete before the experiment		Complete after the experiment	
Planned behavioural experiment	My specific predictions and how much I believe them	Did my predictions come true?	What are my conclusions?

Yes but … This Is My Baby: It Feels Too Risky to Do Things Differently

You might be thinking the stakes just feel too high to do things differently when it involves taking a risk with your baby. Try to remind yourself that you aren't going to be doing anything more risky than the average careful pregnant mum. Think about the precautions you are taking right now – do they guarantee you and your baby's safety? Is that possible? And what are they actually costing you in terms of your well-being and relationships?

Would you recommend the same precautions to other women? Why or why not? Try to focus on what can be gained by taking some active steps to tackle your anxiety.

Dealing with 'Flash Forwards' and Frightening Images

Sometimes our fears present themselves in the form of frightening images rather than verbal thoughts. For some they can feel quite vivid, as if they are flashing forward in time to the worst-case scenario, and often stop at the point you feel most anxious. Naturally these can feel terrifying, especially if they involve thinking the worst or black and white thinking (i.e. only seeing the negative side). It is important to remember images are not facts – they are a product of your mind, not a given of what will happen, and therefore can be challenged, changed or tuned out of in the same way as thoughts, in order to turn down their intensity or bring in a new perspective. Note that our bodies respond in the way they would if the thing was really happening – hence why we can feel scared watching a horror film even though we know they are actors and the blood is fake.

Rhea was experiencing graphic images like this in relation to her fear around pain and birth being difficult and dangerous. The image would play out like a video in her mind and felt very vivid and clear, as if she was there experiencing everything she feared about birth. It would freeze at a point she was in agony and alone.

For Rhea, the first step in tackling this image was to notice when it popped up and label it for what it was. She reminded herself this was just an image, a reflection of her worst fears, not a given of how things would be for her:

'Right now, I'm having an *image* of being in agony left alone rather than 'I will be in agony alone'.

The worst thing for Rhea about this particular image was being on her own in pain.

It is important to remember that images like this are not premonitions, they are just pictures fueling anxiety in the present, therefore they can be changed to address this.

Rhea then experimented with transforming the image. She used information she had gathered so far about birth to create something less intense and frightening. She tried different approaches – playing the image on past the worst point to when the birth was over and she met her baby, bringing people into the image to help and support her with her pain, imagining herself 'coping' – asking for help, breathing, moving around, accessing pain relief and so on. She was still in pain but less paralysed with fear and she felt more in control. Once she had a more balanced and helpful picture in her mind, she practised rehearsing it so it was easier to access when she needed it.

OVER TO YOU
Transforming Frightening Images

What image pops up when you feel anxious?

What is the worst thing about this image? What do you fear it means? How likely does that feel to you right now (0–100%)?

Do you have any new information that doesn't fit with this idea? Is there an alternative view or other possible outcomes that aren't accounted for in the image that are more likely or balanced? Are there ways you might be underestimating your ability to cope and influence what is happening, or that of other people to help you?

Try to bring the anxious image into your mind. Close your eyes if this feels comfortable and try to immerse yourself in what you can see, hear, smell, feel etc. Now experiment with transforming the image in line with what you know now and other possible scenarios. You could try playing the image on, changing who is there, what is happening or what you are saying or doing. There is no right or wrong answer – it is about focusing on what needs to change for you to feel safer and more in control / able to cope.

Really try and immerse yourself in all your senses in the image – what can you see, hear, feel in your body, smell etc. Once you have an alternative image or mini-film in mind, play it to yourself a few times.

How likely does your feared outcome feel now? (0–100%)
Was there any change?
What did you find out?
What does this tell you about the link between images and how you feel?

Taking the Pressure Off: Dealing with Black and White Thinking, 'Shoulds' and 'Musts'

We talked in Chapter 1 about how a tendency to think in a very rigid all-or-nothing way or put pressure on yourself for things to be a certain way can amplify anxiety, guilt and shame and damage your confidence in yourself when you are pregnant. This is because these emotions can pull you into viewing things in extremes rather than allowing you to see how life is full of shades of grey. These are common habits all of us can fall into, but if your aim is to feel more confident in pregnancy, these emotions will make that harder. If you notice this type of pattern in your thinking, then our section on tackling perfectionism in Chapter 6 should be very helpful to you.

Take a step back to examine your thoughts and see if you can consider any alternatives – here are some examples:

Black and white thinking	Realistic reply
I need to be completely safe or I am in total danger	It is impossible to be 100% safe all the time – no-one is but we all survive
If I don't achieve a vaginal birth then I am a total failure as a mother	What I do and who I am aren't the same thing. Judging my whole worth as a mother on the way I birth isn't fair. I would never judge my friends that way
I should feel nothing but positive feelings about the prospect of motherhood	Mixed feelings during motherhood are normal and to be expected Other people will have mixed emotions but they might not talk about it

Black and white thinking	Realistic reply
I must eliminate all risk	This is an impossible task. I can do my best to follow the guidance and advice I have been given about staying well in pregnancy and my birth options but I accept I can never eliminate all risk in life
I must do better than my mum	Mum's parenting was not all bad and I understand now why she might have struggled. There are things that I would like to try and do differently but I know that I am not my mum and my baby is not me so it is okay for us to find our own way too
If my partner and I feel differently then we must have a bad relationship	We have disagreed on lots of things in the past and still enjoy a positive relationship. It is impossible to agree on everything all the time. We can learn from each other's perspectives
I shouldn't feel this scared – there must be something wrong with me	Feeling anxious about pregnancy, birth or parenting is a normal and human way to feel
If I'm not completely in control then I am out of control	Being in control is on a sliding scale; I can be more or less in control in different situations
Unless I plan for every possibility it will all go wrong	I can do some planning and think about my preferences and the support I might need but trying to prepare for every single scenario is impossible and exhausting. I will be better off practising how to build up my tolerance of uncertainty

Accepting Some Uncertainty

The elements of unfamiliarity, ambiguity and unpredictability of pregnancy and entering into motherhood can leave you feeling uncertain and out of control. For most people, facing the unknown will trigger anxiety because it makes it harder for us to effectively prepare for the future and feel able to control or influence what happens to us. In pregnancy this can feel particularly difficult, as what is about to happen is a major life event that of course matters to you very much and feels important to go well.

Uncertainty is also not something we can escape or avoid in the same way as other more tangible fears, e.g. a social situation or large spider hurtling across your kitchen. So, your thinking tries to eliminate it. This means trying to increase certainty through mentally analysing or 'overthinking' the situation – running through all the possible 'what if's' or more active strategies like repeatedly seeking reassurance or taking other precautions like checking or keeping alert for any changes in how you feel. They may have also made you *feel* more in control and reassured in the moment but have they actually made things safer, more predictable or certain over the longer term? See Chapter 2 on worry for more tips on managing uncertainty.

OVER TO YOU
Building Up Your Tolerance of Uncertainty

You can work on building up your tolerance of uncertainty. Have a think about these questions:

What are the ways you are trying to feel more sure in this pregnancy? E.g. going through all possible outcomes in your mind or preparing for the worst ('what ifs' …)?; asking for reassurance; Googling or researching as much as possible; repeatedly checking or keeping vigilant in some way?

What advantages do these strategies have? How have they helped?

What are the downsides? What do they cost you?

Are there some uncertainties you deal with better in life? How do you approach these differently?

Do you have friends who manage uncertainty well? How do they deal with it? Could you ask them?

Go to Chapter 2 on worry for information on techniques to tackle this.

A Note on Monitoring Your Baby's Movements and Home Doppler Kits

If you are more than 28 weeks pregnant, you have likely been advised to start to monitor your baby's movements and get to know their regular pattern so you can spot any changes that might signal they are unwell. Of course, you may have been tracking these earlier too.

If you are already anxious naturally, this can feel like a minefield, as here you are being handed responsibility for checking that your baby is okay – how much movement is enough? What is too little? Too much? What does regular mean? What does a change in movement feel like? What if I miss something? What is meant to help you feel more empowered and confident can actually end up making you feel more anxious and stuck in a cycle of more and more checking and reassurance seeking.

If you are struggling with excessive anxiety about your baby's movements, here are some tips which may help:

- Remember there is no set number of movements you should feel each day or in a certain time frame, as every baby is different.
- You will likely start to notice your baby move between 18 and 24 weeks of pregnancy. It can be later (after 20 weeks) if this is your first pregnancy and a little earlier if this is a subsequent pregnancy. A regular pattern is easier to spot after 28 weeks.
- Movements can feel like a flutter, kick, swish, jab or roll. These typically become more obviously 'kick like' as your pregnancy progresses.
- Get to know your baby's usual pattern of movements by spotting times when they are more active – you may find it useful to chart their movements for a day or two to help you spot a pattern – are there certain times of day or activities which seem to correlate with more movement, e.g. early in the morning, when you are driving, having a bath, lying in a certain position, after eating or drinking something cold etc.? There are apps which can help you to do this.

- Use the times of day and activities you have spotted to help you keep track of your baby's movements at the same time or during the same activity each day. Try to stick with focusing on your baby's movements during these windows of time or activities rather than trying to monitor every single movement every single day.
- NHS advice is **not** to use a home doppler kit to try and check your baby's heartbeat as they are not reliable.
- If your baby's movements feel different or you are concerned, talk to your midwife or maternity unit as soon as you can.

Yes but ... My Pregnancy *Is* High Risk

There is a degree of risk in every pregnancy. However, if you have been told your pregnancy is 'high risk', perhaps because of a pre-existing medical condition, one that develops in pregnancy or previous obstetric complications, it is natural to feel anxious and possibly get drawn into being extra vigilant and so on. All of the exercises we have discussed so far are still relevant to you. Watch out for unhelpful thinking patterns (e.g. jumping to conclusions or all-or-nothing thinking), hypervigilance, repeated reassurance seeking or seeking certainty, unproductive worry and rumination, and avoidance of situations or activities which you have been told are okay. Try to keep in mind that how likely you *feel* it is that something bad will happen is often much higher than the actual risk, even in a higher risk pregnancy. For example, if you have experienced a pre-term birth in a first pregnancy, the risk of a recurrent pre-term labour is around 30%. So, not insignificant, yet often if you are anxious the risk will *feel* much higher than this. Try to gently remind yourself that your feelings are not always a reliable guide to what will happen. Higher risk pregnancies mean a great number of antenatal appointments and certain guidance and recommendations of how to take care of yourself and your baby. Try to stick to what is asked of you rather than doing more than necessary, as this will only fuel your anxiety and make what might feel like a difficult pregnancy harder. Anxiety is something you *can* work on.

Disengage from Worry and Rumination

As we noted earlier, pregnancy-specific anxiety can often trigger worry about how things might go wrong or rumination on past experiences which seem to fit with your fears. Both tend to involve streams of repetitive thoughts that keep you stuck in your head and focused on your fears – they act a bit like 'mental magnets', pulling your attention back onto worst-case scenarios. For more tips and exercises on dealing with excessive worry, take a look Chapter 2.

Bringing Compassion to Your Feelings

If you are struggling with pregnancy-specific anxiety, you may have noticed a tendency to speak to yourself in a harsh and critical way about how you are feeling, e.g. 'What is wrong with me?'; 'Why do I feel so bad?'; 'Will I be able to love my baby?'; 'Am I a terrible person?'. You may see your anxiety as a sign of weakness or failing in some way. Our inner critic can really start to thrive during motherhood. This is particularly common if you tend to take a perfectionistic or all-or-nothing approach to things (see 'Taking the Pressure Off' earlier in this chapter and also tips for tackling perfectionism in Chapter 9 on adjusting to motherhood) and can really add pressure and extra guilt and shame to an already difficult time.

Taking a more compassionate view is not about pitying yourself or giving up on feeling differently. It is about committing to trying to be more accepting, validating the feelings that are accompanying your journey to motherhood, and looking for ways to support and care for yourself when you are struggling, in the same way you would want to be compassionate towards a friend who was finding things difficult.

So, the next time you notice that you're judging yourself for feeling anxious, frustrated or a bit disconnected from your baby, gently remind yourself that you are not alone – that these are common experiences, part of being human, and practise letting them be. Can you think about a kinder way of talking to yourself? Perhaps there is someone you know who might embody a warmer, wiser, more caring approach to your feelings right now. Can you imagine them in your mind's eye? What would they say? How would they sound? What would they do for you? How could you practise taking a more compassionate approach to your feelings and reminding yourself of the value in this? Are there things you would say to yourself or do differently, compared to what you say or do now?

Connecting with Your Baby in Pregnancy

Remember any relationship takes time to develop, including with your baby, and your emotions may not feel particularly strong to begin with. Anxiety can also get in the way of this. If you would like to try and build more of a connection with your baby in pregnancy, below are some gentle things you can try. Start with what feels manageable and realistic now. If you have experienced trauma and find any of these things trigger those memories, it may be helpful to revisit the 'Then versus Now' exercise.

- Talking to, massaging or touching your bump (perhaps with your partner if you have one or another support person) – your baby can hear your voice from 16 weeks, perhaps even earlier
- Responding to your baby's movements with your voice or touch.
- Singing to your baby or enjoying music together
- Visualising you and your baby together once they are born – what would you like to do with them? How would you like to support and parent them? Imagine – what would this look like?
- Making time each day to be alone with your baby somewhere calm and soothing
- Looking at scan pictures or videos from scans
- Consider a 3D or 4D (3D images moving in real time) scan to help have a clearer picture of your baby
- Consider if knowing the gender of your baby may help (or not)
- Preparing or buying things for your baby
- Carrying an item or object with you that represents your baby that you can touch and hold, e.g. baby socks or a muslin

To Sum Up

- Pregnancy-specific anxiety can cover a range of concerns, from your and your baby's health to fears about labour and birth
- Working out your specific fears can help you understand where they come from, and can help you seek reliable information
- Working on other anxiety-maintaining processes such as attention biases, avoidance, excessive reassurance, changing difficult imagery and reducing self-criticism can help

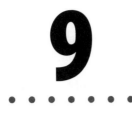

Anxiety and Adjusting to Motherhood

In this chapter you will learn:

➤ What to expect emotionally as you adjust to life after birth
➤ Practical tips on finding your own way as a parent
➤ How to manage worries about being an 'anxious parent'

Adjusting to Parenthood: 'Matrescence'

The early weeks and months after you have your baby are a hugely de-manding time on many fronts. There are further physical changes to pos-sibly navigate (e.g. hormones, pain, bleeding, sometimes incontinence) alongside your recovery from birth. Emotionally, you may feel like you are riding a constant 'rollercoaster' of highs and lows whilst you try to find your feet and adjust to the demands of caring for a newborn who is uniquely dependent yet continuing to rapidly grow and change. Many refer to this time as your baby's unofficial 'fourth' trimester but it is also your first trimester as a new parent and if this is your first baby, a time of building your new identity as a mother.

Even though you have been with your baby for many months during pregnancy, have prepared to meet them and have got through the experience of childbirth, the realities of figuring out new tasks, adapting to a whole new routine and lifestyle, accepting changes to your body and identity (whilst you try to function on minimal sleep) can naturally feel hugely anxiety provoking, perhaps even overwhelming at times. You might struggle to recognise yourself. Suddenly everything can feel uncertain, unpredictable and unknown. Trying to manage so much when you have so little left in the tank can be hugely intense and stressful.

'Matrescence' is a way of thinking about the transition to motherhood. It emphasises that becoming a parent is a process that takes time, from pregnancy or even beforehand, to well into the postnatal period, something like the process of earlier life transitions such as adolescence. Life after birth marks the next chapter in this journey and, just like pregnancy, can continue to feel fraught with mixed emotions – you might feel moments of love and deep connection with your baby, but at other times you might also feel frustrated and trapped and feel a sense of loss for your old life. It can feel simultaneously like the best and hardest thing you have ever done. There might also be panic that your whole identity has now been taken over by being a parent (which it hasn't – see our tips below). You may not have been able to talk about this with others, and you might worry that you aren't feeling the 'right way' and expect better from yourself. This is especially hard in societies (particularly Western culture) which don't fully acknowledge or support women through the process of becoming a mother. It is really important to gently remind yourself that these mixed feelings are a normal part of the adjustment process to becoming a parent – they are part of being human and part of being a mother. Parenting is a hugely challenging job and involves a steep learning curve as you find your way. Feeling conflicted is not a sign that you are a bad parent or do not want or love your baby.

OVER TO YOU
Getting More Information

If you feel that you are not 'getting it right', or not getting motherhood quickly enough, you could consider an experiment to check this out further:

Are there some trusted friends with children who you could ask about their 'matrescence'?

What does your anxiety predict your friends will say about the emotions they experienced as they adjusted to caring for a newborn? How likely does this feel (0–100%)? (E.g. they will all say 'happiness', 100%)

What would you need to ask them to find out?
What did they say?
How does this fit with your prediction?
How does this fit with your view of how the world of new parenting 'should' work?
What have you learnt?

Anxiety as You Navigate Multiple Opinions on Parenting

One thing almost guaranteed for new parents is that they will receive wanted and unwanted advice from multiple sources. Unfortunately, this may not always be consistent. With lots of attention focused on your baby, you may face constant input about 'the best' way to care for them, making it hard to build your confidence and trust your own judgement. Getting stuck in a cycle of doubting yourself and seeking more and more reassurance from books, web searches and other parents, only to be left more confused, is not uncommon. Do I feed on demand or try and get the baby into a routine? Do I give her a dummy or will I be storing up problems for later? Or you might be left thinking you have failed if you try and follow certain 'advice', only to discover it doesn't work or doesn't fit with what your baby wants to do.

Try to remember there is no *right* routine to follow, there is no 'right' way of feeding your baby, getting them to sleep or soothing them. The 'best' start for your baby is what works for you and your family – the method that creates the least stress and greatest chance of happiness and well-being for you both is key – and only you and your baby can be the experts in that. Of course, like any new challenge, finding out what works for you only happens by trial and improvement, so if something isn't working well try not to be hard on yourself and remember, as with any new challenge, your confidence grows the more you do.

If you have a tendency to try to please others or to subjugate your opinion, this is an opportunity to do things differently. You may find the section on 'Self-critical Thinking' in Chapter 6 helpful. You know your baby better than anyone, and your judgement on what makes them happy, safe and well is better than anyone else's. Sometimes you might want someone to make a decision for you – when you are so tired and spent that you can't think straight. That's fine – you can decide to give the responsibility to your partner or other family member and give yourself a break. Remember that you have the right to disagree with others.

If you are finding yourself stuck in a loop of uncontrollable worry about how to parent and paralysed about what decisions to make, then you may find Chapter 2 on worry helpful.

Anxiety from Trying too Hard to Control the Uncontrollable

After birth, so much can feel unpredictable it is natural to want to regain a sense of control. Some things you will be able to influence, e.g. when you go out for a walk and the route you take (although you still might go out hours after your original plan, following an endless cycle of unexpected nappy changes, extra feeds, going back to get something you forgot, changing your own clothes as they have sick on ... etc.!), what your baby wears, what you will have for lunch and dinner and so on, but other things will be more difficult to fully control. Three areas mums often struggle with in this respect are their baby's patterns of feeding, sleeping and crying. Just when you feel you have cracked it, everything can change and feel difficult again. Babies are consistently inconsistent on all these fronts because like any person their appetites, sleep cycles and moods will fluctuate and vary because of a range of different factors, not least because of the massive developmental leaps they will make frequently throughout their first year of life.

It can be easy to fall into the trap of blaming yourself and something you have or haven't done for a tricky period of sleeplessness, fussy during feeding, crying or clinginess, e.g. 'If only I could sort out his naps he would sleep through the night'; 'If I had just winded her better she wouldn't be so cranky'; 'I'm clearly messing up her "latching on" for her to be this fussy feeding'. These ideas can then pull you into greater and greater efforts to get things 'right' – you might find yourself continuously monitoring every minute your baby sleeps and feeds, the time they are awake, trying to catch exactly what happens each time they cry, reviewing the minutiae of your day, to work out what might have gone 'right' or 'wrong' and so on. Of course, sometimes you might spot a solution that helps you to problem solve usefully, but more often than not you will simply end up more and more preoccupied and anxious, as ultimately what you do or don't do is only a part of what is influencing your baby at any one time. If you have noticed yourself feeling very preoccupied and anxious about these issues, try to spot if you might be trying too hard to control what ultimately isn't fully in your control. Are you able to remind yourself of that and experiment with 'loosening the reins' to see if less monitoring and checking help you to feel better?

Anxiety Through Lack of Self-care and Loss of 'You'

Attending to your own needs or asking for help if you are struggling can also feel difficult amidst the societal, or inner, pressure to 'hold it together' and 'get on and enjoy your baby'. It might seem 'selfish' or 'lazy' to take time for yourself, or you might worry that by doing this you are neglecting your baby in some way. It might also just feel impossible to make time in the day, or pointless as you feel you are 'robbing Peter to pay Paul' if you take time out, that you will 'pay for it' later. Consequently, even just looking after the very basics of eating, drinking and resting enough, may fall to the bottom of the pile of priorities. The difficult thing is if your basic needs aren't met and your resources are very low, then the demands of parenting will be much harder to meet and this will only confirm anxious thoughts about your capabilities as a parent. Alternatively, you might feel like your own needs are being pushed aside, which can lead to feelings of anger and frustration.

Making time for your own needs is an essential part of managing your well-being after birth, even if you only look for very small opportunities each day to begin with. It will help to build your resilience and reduce your risk of parental burnout. Neglecting yourself only means your health, relationships (including with yourself and your baby) and your ability to get tasks done will suffer. You might focus on the basics such as brushing your hair and teeth, taking a shower, drinking more water, having tasty snacks in the cupboard or putting on clean clothes first. But it is also important to think about nurturing the other parts of your identity – perhaps the part that enjoys connection with others, being creative, your spiritual side, being physically fit and active and so on.

OVER TO YOU
Reconnecting With What Matters to You

What basic needs, activities or parts of yourself have been neglected or put on hold since the birth of your baby?

What would you like to reconnect with? Try not to focus too much on how possible this feels right now – simply think about what you would like to be doing more of.

What is the very first step you could take towards one of these things today? Who could support you to make this happen?

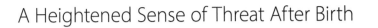

A Heightened Sense of Threat After Birth

After birth your body may feel like it is constantly 'wired' and on high alert. You might notice tension and tightness in your chest or times when your heart seems to race. Some of these sensations might feel unnerving or frightening if they are new and there is no way of explaining them. It's not surprising that your body feels strange as it is undertaking the task of adjusting from your pregnant body to your postnatal body – there is a lot to sort out!

If you find that these sensations then escalate into a panic attack, you will find more information on how to tackle anxious thoughts about body sensations in Chapter 5 on panic.

You may simply feel a general sense of dread that something bad could happen at any moment. The new responsibility of caring for a vulnerable newborn when you lack confidence in your capabilities as a parent can make the stakes feel especially high. As we spoke about in Chapter 3, experiencing unwanted intrusive thoughts or images about harm coming to your baby in these early days is a near universal experience. If these thoughts are worrying you or pulling you into time-consuming rituals of checking and second guessing yourself, the strategies detailed in Chapter 3 should be helpful to you. Remember, thoughts and feelings are not the same as actions, and that 'you are not your thoughts.'

Criticising Yourself into Anxiety

A tendency to be critical and hard on yourself as you adjust to your new role as a mother is also very common. The gap between your 'ideal' self and your reality might be huge. You might notice a constant stream of 'shoulds', 'musts' and 'if onlys' or beat yourself up for being 'such a mess.'

> 'If only I did things more like X, breastfeeding would be going so much better'

'A happy baby should never cry'

'We have waited so long for this, I should always feel happy and grateful'

'I must not feed or rock my baby to sleep, otherwise I am making a rod for my own back'

'The house should always be clean and tidy!'

You might feel preoccupied with the idea there is a 'right way' to parent, to make sure you do things differently to your own parents, or you might feel convinced you are always missing the mark as you doom scroll the endless false realities of social media or compare yourself with the other parents who appear to be 'nailing it'. See the section on setting impossibly high standards in Chapter 6 for some ways to avoid falling into a trap of striving for perfection and focusing on what you perceive as 'inadequacies', and instead take a fairer, less all-or-nothing approach to your parenting abilities. Find a way to approach yourself and your baby with more compassion, so you can accept that a 'good' parent is a 'good enough' parent.

Am I Bonding Enough?

Building a relationship with your baby is like any other relationship in life. It can take time to develop, there is no set 'formula' to getting it right and it will continue to grow and change over time. Feelings of love and connection grow out of getting to know another person and that can take a while, especially when newborn life feels mostly like basic survival very often!

The quality of your future relationship does not depend on the first moments of laying eyes on one another. Unfortunately, women are too often led to believe that after the marathon of childbirth, hormones will kick in and a transcendent moment of otherworldly love will come to pass, followed by endless happiness and satisfaction. Very often this just simply isn't the case, and leaves women vulnerable to feelings of shame and disappointment. Of course, if you have suffered a traumatic labour or birth or had to be separated from your baby after birth, then it is even more understandable that your experience will dampen your emotions (see Chapter 7 on trauma if you feel you continue to be affected by a traumatic birth). Would it surprise you to know that in one study, 40% of first-time mothers and 25% of mothers of two or more children reported 'indifference' as their predominant emotion when meeting their baby? It is a common experience. As with most relationships, 'love at first sight' is the exception, not the rule. It does not make you a bad or uncaring mother and it certainly doesn't mean you are incapable of love for or connection with your child. Simply put, it doesn't matter how you felt when you met your baby. Both you and your baby will build the connection between you.

Connecting With Your Baby After Birth

Babies have an innate need to connect and communicate with you, and over time these early interactions between the two of you will help to shape their brain development. They have a rich vocabulary of cries, movements and facial expressions to express their feelings and needs, but it can often feel difficult and bewildering as a new parent to understand and spot these cues and what your baby might be trying to tell you.

In the following, we give some suggestions of things you can try, to gently build a relationship with your baby after birth. Remember, there is no one correct way to parent, and definitely more than one healthy way to raise a child. What is most important is that you get to know your baby and find ways to be together that work for you both.

It is worth remembering that different babies will have different temperaments, in the same way that different mothers have different personalities. Some babies will be easier to soothe than others, some are very alert and social whilst others take longer to warm up. You might feel you and your baby's personalities complement each other well, e.g. you are both laid back and easy going. But sometimes you might feel there is less of a good fit between the two of you and this can stir up anxiety, e.g. you might be more introverted and shy whereas your baby may seem more extroverted, loud and excitable, which consequently triggers feelings of self-consciousness for you (see Chapter 6 if this is the case for you).

An important note: If you find any of the suggestions below result in the trigger of a vivid or upsetting memory of a traumatic experience, then it may be helpful to look at the 'Then versus Now' exercise in Chapter 7 on trauma, for ideas on how to manage this.

- Allow yourself time to observe your baby and get to know their unique personality
- Try to remain open and curious about your baby as an individual, little person – the more you observe them, the quicker you will get to know their own signs of trying to show you something, e.g. turning their head from side to side or sucking their fist when they are hungry
- Your new baby will enjoy making eye contact with you and you mimicking their expressions
- Try to remember that if your baby looks away whilst they are 'talking' with you, they are not rejecting you – like any of us, they may just need a little break
- Be led by your baby – when they are very little, social interaction can feel quite intense for them, so they may only be able to manage small bursts of 'chatting' with you
- What feels like too much or too little interaction will vary from baby to baby and depend on their temperament. You know your baby best – allow yourself time to find a rhythm which works for both of you. Sometimes the two of you will want to be boisterous and energetic; sometimes cuddly and close; sometimes to have some space
- When you are chatting with your baby, you can talk about what you are thinking, feeling or what you think they might be feeling. They will find this reassuring. 'It's a sunny day today – hooray!'
- You can also talk about what you notice together around you and what you notice them doing; 'I can hear the kettle boiling! Tea for mummy!'; 'Are you playing with your toes?'
- If anxiety means you have been avoiding being with your baby, you could try an experiment to spend a bit more time with them so you have an

opportunity for connection, even if just for a short while. Aim to do this without distractions – try turning off the TV and leaving your phone in another room

- Try holding your baby close – a sling can be helpful, or you can try skin-to-skin contact if that feels manageable for you. However, you don't need to be in 24/7 contact with your baby for their well-being. A baby's 'attachment' to you is not contingent on physical contact – it is more about them having an overall sense of being loved, connected with and cared for

- Gently massaging or bathing your baby can be an enjoyable way to connect with them

- If it feels manageable, you might want to consider a relaxing class that focuses on both your needs, e.g. mother and baby yoga or pilates, or singing together (go for one that includes biscuits!)

- Try not to worry about specific toys and games when your baby is very little – your face, smile and voice are their best first 'toys'

- As your baby grows, they will begin to show more interest in exploring the world around them – they may make playful noises, point, or try to show you things. Think about it like a game of throw and catch or a to and fro – responding to what they are trying to tell you will help to strengthen your relationship

- Try to look out for and spot moments of connection in photos and videos, however fleeting they might seem – making eye contact, looking together, smiling at each other if your baby is older etc. – these moments are evidence of your developing relationship

- Try to remember that crying is your baby's only way of communicating a need – they are not trying to annoy you or being attention seeking. They want to connect with you. If you feel overwhelmed, it is okay to put your baby down somewhere safe and take a few minutes out. Ask for support from someone you trust if you need to

- Try not to worry about the way you feed your baby and its impact on bonding. You can connect with your baby whether you breast, chest, tube or bottle feed (or a combination) by holding your baby close and making eye contact. The best way to feed your baby is the way that creates least stress for you both and allows you to enjoy one another's company

If you feel you need some additional help in bonding with your baby, talk to your health care provider, health visitor and / or family doctor. In the UK, specialist support can usually be found within your local community perinatal mental health team and sometimes your local children's centre. The Parent-Infant Foundation (www.parentinfantfoundation.org.uk) also has details of all the specialist parent–infant teams around the UK, and can help to connect you with the support you feel you need. The Association for Infant Mental Health also provides some excellent resources to help you get to know your baby (www.aimh.uk). We have also added some additional resources at the end of the book. In the US, www.postpartum.net has good resources.

Worries About Being an Anxious Parent and 'Transmitting' Anxiety

Many people seek CBT for anxiety problems because they want to be the best parents they can be and raise confident children, but are worried that this will be difficult due to anxiety. The main thing this shows is that anxious parents care a lot, and our own research shows that this creates a situation in which children feel loved [1]. We know that it is very possible to be an excellent parent and still have anxiety and, furthermore, there are specific things you can do to avoid any impact of anxiety on your child. These include understanding how anxiety works for you and doing as much as you can to help yourself.

If you remembered that you were given some unhelpful messages as a child about yourself or how the world works, think about the messages you would like your own child to pick up. We know that 'modelling', that is, what is actually shown and said to children, is more important than what parents feel on the inside. So, the message is don't worry if some things still make you feel anxious – try to play the role of a confident parent as much as possible, and that is what your child will see. If there are tasks you find difficult due to your own anxiety, if you can, get help to do them rather than avoid doing them altogether. See *Timid to Tiger: Raising Confident*

Kids by Professor Sam Cartwright-Hatton, for an excellent practical guide on parenting with anxiety.

Anxiety in the Context of Covid-19 and Other Social Issues

Being pregnant and looking after a small baby is difficult in the best of situations, but when there is a huge event or series of events that affects the whole of society, this adds unique pressure and difficulties. The years of the Covid-19 pandemic have allowed researchers to gather information about the impact of a variety of stressors on pregnant women and those looking after small children. We will discuss the impact of this, as clear information has emerged on the negative effect of the pandemic. Women have been disproportionately affected by the socioeconomic inequality and economic instability, with more women than men losing their jobs, being unable to source childcare, bearing the brunt of domestic labour and at times educating children. Women are much more likely than men to work causally, meaning that when national lockdowns struck, many women were unable to access wage protections, sickness or maternity pay. Many women found themselves in the position of being the sole carer, performing the lion's share of domestic labour and at times having to take on the role of teacher when homeschooling as well.

Unfortunately, rates of domestic violence and abuse are very high in general, affecting 27% of women aged 15–49 who have been in a relationship, according to the World Health Organization. Rates are known to rise in the context of societal disasters and this has certainly been the case under Covid-19. This may be due to increased time spent with the abuser, increased alcohol use and increased stress on families. This of course increases symptoms of anxiety, depression and trauma in survivors – see the Resources section for more information on where to get help and support if this is relevant to you.

It is clear that a destabilised environment has an impact on everyone across society, but some specific issues have affected pregnant and postnatal women. Women have not been able to access the same support while caring for babies, older children and themselves at this time, as well as being cut off from friends and other networks of informal support. This will increase stress and loneliness.

The Covid-19 pandemic was related to a new transmissible virus. There was considerable uncertainty at the start of this pandemic as to the effect of the virus on pregnant women and their babies, which of course raised anxiety for many. This was stressful for women and their partners, and some people with existing concerns about contamination felt particularly worried.

The circumstances of being separate from partners for scans and labour took away the support that pregnant women rely on in these situations, and probably as a result of all of the above factors, research studies consistently highlighted increased rates of anxiety, stress and traumatic experiences, as well as depression in pregnant women and postnatal mums.

How the Pandemic May Have Impacted Anxious Thoughts and Behaviours and What to Do About it

We have been working with pregnant and postnatal women throughout the Covid-19 pandemic, and during times where other health issues have been prevalent, such as swine flu, ebola and zika virus, which although were not local to our population, did cause worry. There are always a range of responses to any given situation. The key message is that the principles of understanding and fighting anxiety remain the same, and we would encourage you to do what you can to stick to these, within the constraints of your current situation. The techniques of identifying the thoughts and behaviours which are driving anxiety, such as reassurance seeking, checking etc., and then trying to change these, apply whatever the context. Below are some specific issues that have arisen during the Covid-19 pandemic, and what women have found helpful in overcoming anxiety.

Anxious thought / behaviour	What you need to do
Everyone else is worried about contamination, my behaviours are justified	Work out what is average and excessive for this situation and target avoidance, reassurance etc.
My anxiety in social situations is better because I'm not seeing anyone	Compensate for restrictions as much as you can – see people online, outside etc. to test out your anxious thoughts and change self-focus. Try and extend your comfort zone as much as possible with the number, type and situation that you see people in
What if my partner can't be with me during a scan or labour? What if things go wrong and I'm alone?	This may be true due to the social restrictions of the pandemic. Where possible, argue for your partner to be there as much as possible, as this is a protective factor for stress and anxiety later Try and write down any specifics and what you could do Make sure you have charge and data on your phone, reminders of home if in hospital, plans for communication etc.

To Sum Up

- Becoming a parent is a process that can take different amounts of time for people
- Finding yourself as a parent means navigating advice and gaining confidence that you are the best placed person to decide what works
- Parents who have, or are experiencing, anxiety can be excellent parents – tackling your own anxiety as much as possible will be most helpful to you and your family
- Women are often dealing with lots of stressors and these may need to be addressed first before working on anxiety if it is still there

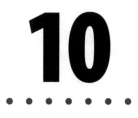

Beyond the Perinatal Period: Taking Your New Skills Forward into Parenthood

Throughout this book we have highlighted ways you can make sense of how anxiety works for you, and start to work on it. The key ideas we have presented are:

➤ Anxiety is a normal and common part of pregnancy and parenthood
➤ When anxiety feels excessive and like it is getting in the way of life, it needs your attention
➤ Anxiety can make us feel in danger, even when we aren't
➤ Feelings of anxiety are never good evidence on their own for what is actually happening (or going to happen)
➤ Behind anxious feelings lie anxious thoughts or the meanings you attach to a particular situation
➤ Working on your anxious thoughts can change how you feel
➤ Anxious thoughts draw you into taking extra precautions to try and feel safer but they only keep anxiety going – they create more problems than they solve

➤ Experimenting with doing things differently is key to breaking this cycle

In this section we want to encourage you to think about what you have learnt so far and how you can take forward what you have achieved and build on it as you navigate the next phases of parenthood. Remember that your anxiety can be worked on and improved by consistently applying these ideas. It's always worth doing even if it is not easy at times and challenging your anxiety is something to be proud of.

---

1. What difficulties have you been working on and how have they been affecting the different areas of your life?

For example:

The main difficulty I have been working on is repeated frightening thoughts and pictures about something bad happening to my baby which come into my mind without warning.

They have made me incredibly anxious and distressed and stopped me from enjoying my baby and doing the things I hoped to do with him. I have been irritable with my partner, friends and loved ones and at times I have felt very alone and depressed.

2. What have you learnt that helps you understand why these difficulties are understandable and not your fault?

For example, I have learnt that:

- *Unwanted intrusive thoughts are very common after having a baby – almost all women experience them*
- *Having a baby is a time full of uncertainty and new challenges and responsibilities which is naturally anxiety provoking*
- *Having a baby is physiologically challenging – the changes in hormones, pain and lack of sleep I was experiencing would have added to my anxiety*
- *I have had some past experiences which mean I find it difficult to tolerate uncertainty and am prone to thinking the worst of myself or putting too much pressure on myself to get things 'just right'*

3. What anxious thoughts have you identified which have kept your difficulties going (Theory A) and what alternative ways of thinking have you been working on (Theory B)?

Were there any general thinking patterns you spotted which trip you up?

For example:

Theory A (what the anxiety tells me)	Theory B (my alternative more helpful perspective)
Your thoughts mean you are a terrible mum who is going to harm their baby	*As I am a loving mother, it is understandable I notice horrible thoughts and they make me feel bad and anxious - however everyone has thoughts they don't want, so this doesn't mean anything about me as a person*

The thinking patterns which don't help me and which I need to be on the lookout for are:

- *Thinking in a very black and white way, e.g. mothers should be perfect*
- *Magical thinking, e.g. having a bad thought means it is more likely to happen*
- *'Shoulds' and 'musts, e.g. I should never have a horrible thought when I'm with my baby and I must immediately attend to their every need to make sure I'm a good mother'*

4. What strategies or precautions have you spotted which have kept your difficulties going and what are the alternative more helpful ways of doing things?

For example:

Old strategies	New strategies
Never be alone with my baby	*Experiment with being with my baby on my own even if I have the thoughts*
Work hard to push the thoughts away	*Treat the thoughts as thoughts – allow them to come and go*
Don't tell anyone about the thoughts	*Talk about the thoughts and how upsetting they have been – seek support*

5. What key things have you found out or learnt from working on your unhelpful thoughts and behaviours?

For example:

- *How I feel is not a reliable guide to what actually happens*
- *The more I monitor myself for signs of danger the more anxious I feel*
- *Other people have intrusive thoughts too – I am not alone*
- *People sympathise and haven't shamed me*
- *Not doing what I usually do does mean I feel anxious but I can tolerate it and it does eventually subside*

6. What are the key techniques which have helped you?

For example:

- *Experimenting with doing things differently*
- *Evaluating the evidence for what I believed my thoughts meant about me*
- *Asking for support not reassurance*
- *Prioritising rest when I can*

7. What changes have you made since you started working on your anxiety? What progress have you made towards your goals?

For example:

- *I can now be alone with my baby and not feel terrified*
- *I am less afraid of my thoughts and able to let them go*
- *I am seeking less reassurance and asking for a different kind of support*

8. How do you want to take this forward? What are your next steps?

For example:

- *I want to take my baby on a trip by myself*
- *I want to try and join a support group for other mums affected by intrusive thoughts like me, so I can share my story and maybe help others*

9. What things might have the potential to trigger more anxiety again in the future?

For example:

- *My baby starting to crawl and do more by himself*
- *Weaning*
- *The stress of starting to back to work and my baby starting nursery*

10.   How would you know you were starting to struggle again? What would be the first signs?

For example:

- *I would be worrying about my thoughts again*
- *I would be questioning my judgement and asking for more reassurance than usual*
- *I would start to avoid situations*
- *I would become more withdrawn*
- *I would feel tearful and not sleep as well*

11.   How would you deal with a setback like this? What would be helpful? What would not be helpful?

For example:

Helpful	Not helpful
Talk to people I trust – ask for support	*Hide how I am feeling*
Read through this section of the book and revisit any chapters which seem helpful	*Repeatedly ask for reassurance*
Confront the situations I am afraid of – set up an experiment	*Avoid things more and more*

Appendices

Appendix 1: Anxiety-informed Birth Planning

Every mum deserves a positive birth experience, but if you are experiencing a lot of anxiety this might feel hard to achieve. Below are some tips and questions to think about ahead of your birth, to ensure looking after your mental health is factored into your plans and the support you are offered.

- Who will be supporting you through the birth of your baby? Include your birth partner, doula, professionals etc. It is important that everyone is well informed about what you might need.
- What is helpful for them to know about the anxiety you have been struggling with? You might consider sharing extracts from this book or notes to help them understand what you need to support you, in addition to your birth plan itself.
- For example, it might be useful for them to know how you tend to respond when you are anxious, e.g. go very quiet, dissociate or perhaps the opposite – feel more agitated and irritable, or ask for reassurance repeatedly, even if you are told things are okay. This way they can help to spot when the temperature is rising on your anxiety, check in with you and take steps to help soothe and support you effectively.
- You could consider a code word or phrase that your birth partner and care team are made aware of to signal you are feeling more overwhelmed.
- Are there particular aspects of birth which you anticipate might be very anxiety provoking or triggering for you? For example, being in pain, lying down, being examined, feeling very hot, bright lights, tearing, or certain words or phrases being said etc.?
- Are there specific fears about what could happen during the birth itself which you have been struggling with, e.g. losing control, your body not being able to do it, being left alone, your baby or you coming to harm?
- As per Chapter 8 on pregnancy-specific anxiety, is there trusted information you can gather from professionals ahead of time, to evaluate how likely these outcomes feel? Ask for an extra appointment with your midwife to discuss these things if useful. How could you have that information easily accessible to you during birth, to remind and reassure you?

- How can care be tailored to support you best and alleviate your anxiety?
- Are there aspects of your physical care and the environment to be considered? For example, would you like early pain relief, minimal vaginal examinations, lights dimmed, music playing, to be able to move around as much as possible or not lie fully flat or prone?
- If you have particular grounding objects, smells, body positions or phrases make sure those supporting you are aware of these.
- What style of communication suits you best when you are anxious – do you prefer space and quiet, or lots of direct encouragement and reassurance? Do you want procedures to be explained to you or would you prefer information is shared another way, e.g. for information to be shared with your birth partner?
- Are there particular words or phrases you find triggering or undermining for your confidence? What could people say instead to support you?
- Are there any other cultural or spiritual considerations which those supporting you should be aware of to help you feel less anxious?
- Even with extensive preparation, birth can still be unpredictable. Watch out for black and white thinking about how you feel birth 'should' be. Remember, whilst there are many choices you can make and things you can influence, some events may still happen outside of your control.
- Try to stay flexible in your thinking and approach birth considering your preferences and the support you might need across different scenarios, e.g if you require more pain relief, need emergency help to birth your baby such as forceps, ventouse or a C-section.
- If you were to have an abdominal birth (C-section), are there any special considerations for those caring for you? Do you have preferences for meeting your baby? E.g., would you like the curtain lowered so you can see your baby being born? To be allowed to discover the baby's sex in your own time etc.?
- Would you like immediate skin-to-skin contact where possible or would you prefer your birth partner to hold your baby?
- What support would you like with infant feeding? Would you like to breast, bottle or combination feed?
- In what way can postnatal care be enhanced to support you? E.g., if you anticipate sharing a space with other women will exacerbate your anxiety whilst you try to get to know your baby, you can request a side room (if available).

Appendix 2: Improving Your Sleep

Disturbed sleep when you are pregnant or have a new baby to care for is of course to be expected. However, the effects of anxiety or trauma and the habits you may have formed around sleep can make it even harder to rest, even if you are able to. E.g., your sleep might be disturbed by nightmares or you might feel afraid to sleep (e.g. if lying down or the dark are possible memory triggers for you); checking for danger (for yourself or your baby) might make it hard to relax into sleep and worry might keep you awake. If you find yourself worrying a lot at night time, you may find the ideas in Chapter 2 on worry helpful.

Additional sleep deprivation when you are already exhausted can feel torturous and only add to feelings of distress and overwhelm. We need sleep for our physical and emotional well-being. However, it is an automatic process – we cannot force it to happen – hence why it is not always helpful to be repeatedly told 'you must sleep when the baby sleeps!' Many of the techniques described in the book so far should help alleviate some of the additional barriers for sleep for you, e.g. the sections on tackling memory triggers, rumination and dissociation. Here we describe some additional specific techniques to help support your body's readiness for sleep.

Good Sleep Hygiene

By good sleep hygiene we mean getting into the habits needed for good-quality night-time sleep (when you are able to!) and day time alertness.

In Pregnancy

- Try to ease reflux symptoms by eating small amounts frequently, prop yourself up in bed or raise the head of the bed if possible
- Lie on your left side and use pillows to support your bump, hips and back
- Try to reduce your fluid intake 2–3 hours before bedtime
- Try to exercise and keep active (as long as not medically contraindicated)
- Avoid all screens half an hour before bed and during the night if you wake up
- Keep bed for sleep and sex only – avoid working or watching TV in bed
- Try to be consistent with your bedtime and getting up time, but try only to go to bed when you feel tired
- Practise some relaxing activities shortly before bed, e.g. stretching, caffeine-free tea, wind-down music

- If you do wake up and struggle to get back to sleep, try a low-stimulus activity until you feel sleepy again, e.g. reading
- If you need to nap in the day, try to keep these earlier in the day if possible

After Birth

- Consider a 'next to me' style crib to help keep feeds and nappy changes as straightforward as possible
- If you are bottle or combination feeding, you may find it helpful to sleep in shifts and have some sleeping time away from your baby, if being in the same room as your baby and partner makes it too difficult to relax into sleep
- Try to practise some relaxing activities shortly before bed, e.g. stretching, a hot shower, caffeine-free tea, wind-down music
- Avoid caffeine and chocolate later in the day and before bed
- If you can, try to get outside into the daylight each day and walk a little – regular exercise can lift your mood and support your readiness for sleep
- Keep your bedroom as dark and quiet as possible when you are trying to sleep. Use a nightlight instead of turning on brighter lights when you need to get up to care for your baby or use the toilet
- Try to avoid screens before bed and in the night if possible
- Ask for support with night-time feeds if you are very exhausted. Consider the benefits of bottle- as well as breastfeeding (or a combination of both) for your mental well-being, if lack of sleep is significantly adding to your distress
- Ask for support in the day so you can reduce your sleep deficit with a nap if possible, but try to avoid napping too close to bedtime
- If you do wake whilst your baby is sleeping and struggle to go back to sleep, try a low-key activity until you feel sleepy again, e.g. reading

Appendix 3: Improving Your Mood when You Feel Depressed

When feeling low or depressed, you may withdraw from, avoid, or simply be unable to do activities which usually give you pleasure or a sense of accomplishment, which can trigger feelings of loss and loneliness. If taking care of your baby means your own needs have been neglected, then it is also natural that feelings of depression might begin to surface. Symptoms of depression include losing interest in things you would usually enjoy, feeling tearful, sad, guilty, worthless, tired, slowed down and hopeless about the future. You may also notice a loss of appetite and libido (interest in sex). Life might feel like it has just become a never-ending series of menial tasks which give you little or no satisfaction – you might feel like you are just 'going through the motions.' If you have given birth, you may struggle to find closeness with your baby or any meaning in motherhood or you may feel desperately alone and that no-one understands. You may feel constantly busy but like nothing is ever achieved.

When you feel tired, lacking in energy and motivation, and feel little pleasure any more, it is natural to become more withdrawn and put off tasks. It can be hard to get going again. Some tasks might feel too tricky or difficult to do or fit into your day. What you need to do and what you feel like doing can be very different. However, we all need meaningful activity to help support our well-being and give us a sense of purpose. Reducing activity keeps depression going. It easily kickstarts a vicious cycle – doing less results in feeling more depressed, less motivated and dwelling on negative ideas about yourself and your future more readily, e.g. 'I'm a failure'; 'I am worthless'; 'I'm useless'; 'I don't deserve to feel happy'; 'Nothing will ever get better'; which then pull your mood and motivation down even further. If you are trying to adjust to the demands of caring for a new baby, you may also find it hard to keep up with meeting even your basic needs regularly (such as eating regularly, getting showered and dressed etc.). Feelings of depression can make that even harder.

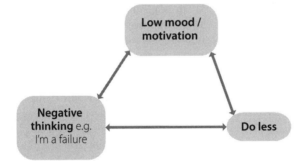

Breaking this cycle means trying to change what you do when you feel low – moving from avoidance into action and asking for help when you need it; challenging negative thinking or expectations of yourself and nurturing yourself as well as your baby. It means making decisions of what to do based on *how you want to feel* (for you and for your baby) rather than how you are feeling right now. It means doing simple things regularly – things which give you a sense of *accomplishment* (e.g. brushing your hair each day, showering each day, putting on clean clothes, getting out of the house each day) *and* things which would usually give you a sense of *pleasure* (e.g. checking in with a friend, listening to some upbeat music, buying yourself some flowers or a magazine, playing with your baby). It also means rec-ognising that your needs are as important as your baby's (and other people's) and sometimes need to be prioritised to enable you to feel better and be the mother you would like to be. Looking after you is not an act of selfishness. It is essential. Think of it like fitting your own oxygen mask first – you cannot do anything for anyone if you run out of oxygen. But also, try to give yourself permission to care for yourself and ask for help because *you* are worthy of your time and care. Because you matter as well as your baby. No-one can do everything by themselves and your identity stretches beyond motherhood.

This may all sound very well in theory but we know it isn't always easy in practice. Doing things differently takes energy, which isn't always in great supply during pregnancy or postnatally. The key is to look out for little opportunities to begin to build pleasure, self-care and a sense of accomplishment back into your day, and focus on how you want to feel rather than what you feel like doing now. Try to make some specific, manageable and realistic plans that you sense you could have a go at a specific time – choose a time of day that you think will offer you the easiest opportunity for change. Remember plans might need to be creative – they might need to involve your baby or it might mean asking for some support from others so you can have some time away from your baby. Sometimes you might need to try things and realise that they don't work out in order to find out what might need to be done differently next time. Try to be gentle with yourself – if things don't work out, see this as an exercise of trial and improvement and try again another time. All we want you to do is have a go at something small you feel you would usually enjoy or might give you a sense of satisfaction. Try things out one step at a time.

Negative thinking such as 'I'm a failure' and 'useless' are common ways of attacking yourself when you are low. It is important to know that these thoughts are a feature of low mood, not facts. Treating these thoughts as facts can make enjoying life and motherhood hard. This in turn becomes further evidence for failing. However, just because you *feel like* a failure does not mean you are. You may have had a lot of ideas about how pregnancy, birth or parenthood might be and now that things are different from what you hoped or expected you may feel you aren't a good enough parent or cut out to be a mum. Society puts a lot of pressure on women to be a certain type of mother – to feel a certain way, have a certain type of birth, feed their baby in a certain way, be able to do it all. It's an unfair expectation that often fuels disappointment and shame. This is not your fault. Are you putting too much pres-sure on yourself, trying to do too much? Are you struggling to ask for help because you feel like you should do it all? Are you trying to live up to some kind of 'super-mum' myth? Are you ignoring your positive qualities or things you have achieved? If the answer to any of these questions is yes then you may find it helpful to look back at our tips on tackling perfectionism in Chapter 9 on adjusting to parenthood.

References and Resources

References

Chapter 1

1. Dennis, C., Falah-Hassani, K., & Shiri, R. (2017). Prevalence of antenatal and postnatal anxiety: systematic review and meta-analysis. *British Journal of Psychiatry*, 210(5), 315–323. https://doi.org/10.1192/bjp.bp.116.187179

2. Arch, J. J., Dimidjian, S., & Chessick, C. (2012). Are exposure-based cognitive behavioral therapies safe during pregnancy? *Archives of Women's Mental Health*, 15, 445–457. https://doi.org/10.1007/s00737-012-0308-9

Chapter 2

1. Glover, V., & Capron, L. (2017). Prenatal parenting. *Current Opinion in Psychology*, 15, 66–70. https://doi.org/10.1016/j.copsyc.2017.02.007

2. Stein, A., Craske, M. G., Lehtonen, A., et al. (2012). Maternal cognitions and mother-infant interaction in postnatal depression and generalized anxiety disorder. *Journal of Abnormal Psychology*, 121(4), 795–809.

3. Challacombe, F., Feldmann, P., Lehtonen, A., et al. (2007). Anxiety and interpretation of ambiguous events in the postnatal period: an exploratory study. *Behavioural and Cognitive Psychotherapy*, 35(4), 495–500.

Chapter 3

1. Fairbrother, N., & Woody, S. R. (2008). New mothers' thoughts of harm related to the newborn. *Archives of Women's Mental Health*, 11(3), 221–229. https://doi.org/10.1007/s00737-008-0016-7

2. Leckman, J., Mayes, L., Feldman, R., et al. (1999). Early parental preoccupations and behaviors and their possible relationship to the symptoms of obsessive-compulsive disorder. *Acta Psychiatrica Scandinavica Supplementum*, 100(Suppl. 396), 1–26. https://doi.org/10.1111/j.1600-0447.1999.tb10951.x

3. Barrett, R., Wroe, A. L., & Challacombe, F. L. (2016). Context is everything: an investigation of responsibility beliefs and interpretations and the relationship

with obsessive-compulsive symptomatology across the perinatal period. *Behavioural and Cognitive Psychotherapy*, 44(3), 318–330. https://doi.org/10.1017/S1352465815000545

4. Fairbrother, N., Collardeau, F., Albert, A. Y. K., et al. (2021). High prevalence and incidence of obsessive-compulsive disorder among women across pregnancy and the postpartum. *Journal of Clinical Psychiatry*, 82(2), 20m13398. https://doi.org/10.4088/JCP.20m13398

5. Guglielmi, V., Vulink, N. C., Denys, D., et al. (2014). Obsessive-compulsive disorder and female reproductive cycle events: results from the OCD and reproduction collaborative study. *Depression and Anxiety*, 31(12), 979–987. https://doi.org/10.1002/da.22234

Chapter 4

1. Ost, L. G., & Sterner, U. (1987). Applied tension: a specific behavioral method for treatment of blood phobia. *Behaviour Research and Therapy*, 25(1), 25–29. https://doi.org/10.1016/0005-7967(87)90111-2

2. Lilliecreutz, C., Josefsson, A., & Sydsjo, G. (2010). An open trial with cognitive behavioral therapy for blood- and injection phobia in pregnant women: a group intervention program. *Archives of Women's Mental Health*, 13(3), 259–265. https://doi.org/10.1007/s00737-009-0126-x

Chapter 7

1. Farren, J., Jalmbrant, M., & Ameye, L., et al. (2016). Post-traumatic stress, anxiety and depression following miscarriage or ectopic pregnancy: a prospective cohort study. *BMJ Open*, 6, e011864. https://doi.org/10.1136/bmjopen-2016-011864

2. Zambaldi, C. F., Cantilino, A., & Sougey, E. B. (2011). Bio-socio-demographic factors associated with post-traumatic stress disorder in a sample of postpartum Brazilian women. *Archives of Women's Mental Health*, 14, 435–439. https://doi.org/10.1007/s00737-011-0224-4

Chapter 8

1. Chandra, P. S., & Nanjundaswamy, M. H. (2020). Pregnancy-specific anxiety: an under-recognized problem. *World Psychiatry*, 19(3), 336–337. https://doi.org/10.1002/wps.20781

2. Nath, S, Lewis, L. N., Bick, D., et al. (2021). Mental health problems and fear of childbirth: a cohort study of women in an inner-city maternity service. *Birth*, 48, 230–241. https://doi.org/10.1111/birt.12532

3. Slade, P., Balling, K., Sheen, K., & Houghton, G. (2019). Establishing a valid construct of fear of childbirth: findings from in-depth interviews with women and midwives. *BMC Pregnancy and Childbirth*, 19(1), 96. https://doi .org/10.1186/s12884-019-2241-7

4. Pearson, R., & Lewis, M. B. (2005). Fear recognition across the menstrual cycle. *Hormones and Behavior*, 47(3). https://doi.org/10.1016/j.yhbeh .2004.11.003

Chapter 9

1. Challacombe, F. L., Salkovskis, P.M., Woolgar, M., et al. (2017). A pilot randomized controlled trial of time-intensive cognitive-behaviour therapy for postpartum obsessive-compulsive disorder: effects on maternal symptoms, mother-infant interactions and attachment. *Psychological Medicine*, 47(8), 1478–1488.

When and How to Seek Professional Help

If you are currently so affected by anxiety that it is hard to function day to day, then it is likely you will benefit from professional support. The ideas presented here may still be helpful to you but are likely to be most effective alongside the help of an appropriately trained therapist. Try to talk to your midwife, obstetrician, doctor or other health professional at the earliest opportunity, so they can help you to access the support available to you in your area.

The right service to meet your needs will depend on your personal circumstances and the complexity of the difficulties you are managing. It is not a decision you need to make alone. It is important you receive help from a therapist with knowledge and understanding (or access to specialist consultancy) of the perinatal context and how this can affect anxiety and vice versa.

There are also many excellent third sector (e.g. charity) organisations offering support. See below for some further resources or visit www.maternalmental healthalliance.org for a directory of support organisations local to you in the UK, or www.mmhla.org if you are in the US.

Selected Resources

(A Complete List Can Be Found Online)

Pregnancy (General)

What to Expect When You are Expecting, by Heidi Murkoff – a comprehensive guide to pregnancy month by month.

www.arc-uk.org – support and information through antenatal testing

Baby Buddy App (www.babybuddy.co.uk) – a multi-award winning interactive pregnancy and parenting guide in an easily accessible app

www.medicinesinpregnancy.org – a useful resource summarising the evidence for the best use of medicines in pregnancy

www.mothertobaby.org – a US resource providing evidence-based information to mothers about medication in pregnancy

www.pregnancysicknesssupport.org.uk/ – support for hyperemesis gravidarum

www.tommys.org – information on many aspects of pregnancy, especially complications, prematurity and miscarriage

Pregnancy and Parenting After Infertility

Precious Babies: Pregnancy, Birth and Parenting after Infertility, by Kate Brian

Pregnancy Loss

Empty Cradle, Broken Heart: Surviving the Death of Your Baby, by Deborah Davis – pregnancy and parenting after loss

When a Baby Dies: The Experience of Late Miscarriage, Still Birth and Neonatal Death, by Alix Henley

www.compassionatefriends.org

www.miscarriageassociation.org.uk – support after miscarriage at any stage of pregnancy

www.sands.org.uk – support after stillbirth and baby loss

Premature and Sick Babies

Intensive Parenting: Surviving the Emotional Journey through the NICU, by Deborah Davis & Mara Tesler Stein

www.bliss.org.uk – charity for babies born premature or sick

www.leosneonatal.org/ – charity for neonatal families during NICU stay or discharge

Adjusting to Motherhood

What No One Tells You: A Guide to Your Emotions from Pregnancy to Motherhood, by Alexandra Sacks & Catherine Birndorf – normalising all the different feelings you may experience as you transition to motherhood

What Mothers Do, by Naomi Stadlen – useful guide to some of the realities of motherhood and how they can clash with expectations

www.parentinfantfoundation.org.uk – connecting parents with support for their relationship with their baby

Postnatal Depression

https://apni.org/ – the association of postnatal illness offering support for anyone affected by postnatal illness

www.postpartum.net – international organisation dedicated to supporting those affected by post-partum mental illness

Post-partum Psychosis

www.app-network.org – national charity for women and their families affected by post-partum psychosis

www.maternalocd.org – support for intrusive thoughts and OCD. Charity founded and run by two women with lived experience of maternal OCD, to raise awareness of the issue amongst professionals and mothers alike

Post-traumatic Stress

www.birthtraumaassociation.org.uk – charity supporting women affected by birth trauma

www.makebirthbetter.org – collective campaigning to reduce the incidence of birth trauma; offers information and signposting to anyone affected

Fathers

www.dadsmatteruk.org – support for dads affected by depression, anxiety or PTSD

Violence and Abuse

Bright Sky App (www.hestia.org/brightsky) – discreet app offering support and information for anyone affected by domestic violence

www.nationaldahelpline.org.uk/ – information, support and freephone helpline for anyone suffering from domestic abuse

www.womensaid.org.uk – support for women and children affected by domestic violence

Maternity Rights

www.birthrights.org.uk – charity supporting women to ensure their rights in pregnancy and childbirth are upheld

Index

Entries in **bold** refer to tables; those in *italic* to figures